The Dissociative Identity Disorder Sourcebook

The Dissociative Identity Disorder Sourcebook

Deborah Bray Haddock,
M.Ed., M.A., L.P.

Foreword by James A. Chu, M.D.

McGraw·Hill

New York   Chicago   San Francisco   Lisbon   London   Madrid   Mexico City
Milan   New Delhi   San Juan   Seoul   Singapore   Sydney   Toronto

Library of Congress Cataloging-in-Publication Data

Haddock, Deborah Bray, 1956–
  The dissociative identity disorder sourcebook / Deborah Bray Haddock.
      p.   cm.
  ISBN 0-7373-0394-8
  1. Multiple personality.   I. Title.

  RC569.5.M8 .H34   2001
  616.85'236—dc21   2001028361

10 11 12 13 14 15 16 17   DOC/DOC   0 9

ISBN 0-7373-0394-8

Cover design by Laurie Young

McGraw-Hill books are available at special quantity discounts to use as premiums and sales promotions, or for use in corporate training programs. For more information, please write to the Director of Special Sales, Professional Publishing, McGraw-Hill, Two Penn Plaza, New York, NY 10121-2298. Or contact your local bookstore.

This book is not intended to be used for the purpose of diagnosing or treating dissociative identity disorder.

In all examples, names and certain specific details have been changed to protect confidentiality.

This book is printed on acid-free paper.

To Milt

Contents

Foreword

 $\mathbf{W}$ e—the community of those who study, treat, or live with dissociative disorders—have been waiting for this book for a long time. *The Dissociative Identity Disorder Sourcebook* is a welcome new addition to the growing literature on the treatment of persons with multiple identities. Deborah Haddock has a gift for being able to explain complex phenomenology in clear and understandable language. Her book provides valuable information to clinicians who are relatively new to the diagnosis and treatment of dissociative identity disorder (DID). Most important, however, is that this book provides welcome guidance to persons with DID.

"Is there anything I can read to help me understand my problems?" I have been asked this question by dozens of people who were beginning their treatment for dissociative difficulties. Other than some first-person accounts and basic booklets, there has been little to recommend to them. The *Dissociative Identity Disorder Sourcebook* is the first resource to describe the genesis of DID and the process of treatment with both simplicity and sophistication. This book is truly appropriate for use by patients, who should pace their reading as tolerated in consultation with their therapists.

The Dissociative Identity Disorder Sourcebook explains the intermix of dissociative and posttraumatic symptoms, difficulties with self-esteem, and relational problems, tracing their roots as adaptive mechanisms that derive from overwhelmingly traumatic experiences. As a result, this book may go a long way to help to destigmatize and depathologize these difficulties, to reduce the secret shame that all childhood abuse survivors suffer, and to explain the experience of persons with DID to a wide audience.

The Dissociative Identity Disorder Sourcebook is written from the patient's perspective and is eminently practical. For example, choosing a therapist is often a huge hurdle, but this book describes all the steps—locating a therapist, dealing with insurance when selecting a therapist, describing the qualities of therapists that are helpful—and the different treatment approaches that therapists may use. I found the information on what is not good or appropriate therapy particularly useful in defining what both patients and therapists need to do to make sure that boundaries of a good therapeutic relationship are established and respected.

The Dissociative Identity Disorder Sourcebook describes the process of therapy, including the phases of treatment, and gives many useful exercises and tools. For example, in the discussion of the critical process of stabilization are many examples of grounding techniques and help on how to set up a basic safety plan. The sections on how to begin work with alter personalities, to share information, and to manage feelings are extremely helpful in beginning the process of treatment. *The Dissociative Identity Disorder Sourcebook* also addresses the dilemmas that inevitably arise in treatment and offers practical advice about how they may be understood and resolved.

Perhaps the strongest theme of this book is its empowering message of hope. Although the treatment of DID is realistically portrayed as long term, treatment is described as possible and doable. The tasks and difficulties in treatment are not minimized, and Deborah Haddock emphasizes patients' active role in treatment beyond just passively accepting nurturance and guidance. It is perhaps this message—that persons with DID must accept responsibility for their problems even though they were induced by others and feel totally outside their control, and that they must strive to trust others to help find solutions to these problems—that is the most important, empowering, and enduring contribution this book can make.

JAMES A. CHU, M.D.
Chief of Hospital Clinical Services,
McLean Hospital
Associate Professor of Psychiatry,
Harvard Medical School
Author, *Rebuilding Shattered Lives*

Preface

As an undergraduate student in psychology, I was taught that multiple personalities were a very rare and bizarre disorder. That is all that I was taught on the subject. Then, many years later, I came to know someone with this supposedly rare disorder, then someone else, and then someone else. It soon became apparent that what I had been taught was simply not true. Not only was I meeting people with multiplicity; these individuals entering my life were normal human beings with much to offer. They were simply people who had endured more than their share of pain in this life and were struggling to make sense of it.

Fortunately, I was in graduate school when I began to explore this phenomenon, and I was given ample opportunity to study and discuss the topic of dissociative identity disorder (DID), which at that time was known as multiple personality disorder (MPD). I researched and wrote about art therapy with MPD, about posttraumatic stress disorder, about the myths associated with MPD, and eventually about how I planned to integrate my newly learned skills in Adlerian therapy into my work with this population. I took workshop after workshop on the topic and obtained supervision from therapists with far more knowledge and expertise than I had. I still continue to learn, as do all therapists in the field of trauma. This discipline is still in its infancy, yet growing by leaps and bounds. And that brings me to my main reason for writing *The Dissociative Identity Disorder Sourcebook*.

As a therapist, I have many avenues in which to learn about DID, but I hear exactly the opposite from clients and others who are struggling to understand their own existence. When I talk to them about the need to let supportive people into their lives, I always get a variation of the same answer. "It is not safe. They won't understand." My goal here is to provide a small piece of that gigantic puzzle of understanding. If this book helps someone with DID start a conversation with a supportive friend or family member, understanding will be increased. If it provides an opportunity for a therapist and client to talk about treatment options or their own personal beliefs surrounding DID, understanding will be increased. Even if someone reads this book believing it will be another sensationalistic story about multiple personalities, understanding will be increased.

I truly believe that as understanding increases, DID will come to be seen as a lifesaving defense. DID is about survival! As more people begin to appreciate this concept, individuals with DID will start to feel less as though they have to hide in shame. DID develops as a response to extreme trauma that occurs at an early age and usually over an extended period of time. Usuually, but not always, the trauma comes in the form of child abuse or neglect. Some people with DID are extremely high functioning in their daily lives; and others experience crises that leave them expending enormous amounts of energy simply trying to cope from day to day. Yet all share similar stories and the hope of a happier and more peaceful life.

As you read the pages that follow, bear in mind that I am speaking to many different people. I often refer to the person with DID as "she" because women are more likely to seek treatment. However, males also have DID and their struggles are no less than those of women. I also use terms such as *dissociative* and *dissociator* when talking about people with DID. This is because I am writing to a large audience and, although it may seem impersonal at times, such wording is the best way to speak to all audiences at once. It is not meant to be discounting in any way. I also use the term *disorder* throughout the book. I struggled with whether to use this term because I did not want to downplay the positive role that dissociation and alternate personalities, or identities, play in the life of someone with DID. This book does, however, address the many difficulties experienced by those who live with dysfunctional dissociation, and it does so in the context of psychological treatment. Within that context it is appropriate to refer to DID as a disorder. My use of that term, however, is neutral and not a judgment on the nature of dissociation. My personal belief about DID is this: It was life saving. It is about survival. And in an individual's posttrauma adult life, it can be both dysfunctional and life affirming at the same time.

In addition to increasing understanding about DID, I also chose to write this book because the shame experienced by those with DID often causes them to suffer in silence. My desire was to write a book for those with DID that would offer clear information without the sensationalism that often accompanies this topic, but that didn't seem to be enough. I realized that the book also needed to be written in such a way that a person significant in the life of someone with DID could begin to understand the world of dissociation as well. After all, shame and secrecy go hand in hand. I also decided to include information for therapists that would address the treatment of DID. My hope was to create a book that could truly be considered a sourcebook, one that could be shared and discussed among an individual with DID and the significant people in her life, including therapists. From my interactions with other mental health professionals, I also know that there is a certain stigma associated with DID that can frighten people away from treating the disorder. This book is also for those therapists, so I like to think of it as an introduction to the treatment and management of DID, a resource that can help demystify dissociation and help people to view it in a more compassionate light.

The overall goal of the book is to provide readers with educational information on the identification, treatment, and management of DID. Each chapter was written to address issues of concern for both laypeople and professionals who are interested in or affected by the phenomena of dissociation. Chapter 1 provides an overview of the topic of dissociation, with an emphasis on DID. It offers a glimpse into the history of dissociation and how it is viewed today. Chapter 2 discusses DID in terms of its development and whether it should be thought of as dysfunction or as an adaptive response to trauma.

Chapters 3 through 5 focus on the diagnosis and treatment of DID. These chapters are written for both the layperson and the professional in the hope that they will help clients with DID become active participants in the treatment process.

Chapter 6 addresses the very real experience of feeling "stuck" in therapy. This chapter talks about ways the disorder itself might be contributing to this problem, but it also talks about why adjunct therapies might be needed. Adjunct therapies addressed include art therapy, eye movement desensitization and reprocessing, dialectical behavior theory, hypnosis, and bodywork. The use of medication in conjunction with therapy is addressed in chapter 7; chapter 8 provides an introduction to group therapy and discusses why it might be helpful.

Chapter 9 is addressed to individuals with DID and offers self-help and coping strategies that can be put to immediate use. In chapter 10 the focus is on the friend, family member, therapist, or other supportive person in the life of someone with DID. This chapter talks about boundaries, communication issues, and self-care.

The epilogue includes parting thoughts and is followed by appendices that offer valuable information about inpatient treatment options, books and other resources, and Internet sites. The information provided will be helpful for anyone wanting to learn more about DID.

Caution: As you begin to read this book, remember that even educational material can bring up many feelings. Also, the personal stories about trauma and dissociation included in these chapters may encompass material that is triggering for some people. If you are easily triggered, do not read personal accounts when you are alone. If, for any reason, you begin to experience emotion that feels overwhelming, it is probably an internal signal that you need to put the book away until a later time. Please respect the pace at which you can process this information. As you begin reading, I hope you do so in the spirit of personal growth for you and you alone.

Acknowledgments

I gratefully acknowledge Bud Sperry and the people at Contemporary Books for giving me the opportunity to write about something that is important to me. Most important, I thank Peter Hoffman for so graciously adopting a work in progress, Hudson Perigo for her encouraging feedback, and Rena Copperman, my managing editor.

My heartfelt appreciation also goes to:

- Those people I have known throughout the years who have struggled with dissociation in a world where most people simply do not understand.
- My colleagues throughout the world who are working diligently to advance the treatment of DID, yet who still found the time to read for me, offer feedback, complete surveys, and answer many, many questions in my quest for a deeper knowledge and understanding of this topic. Special thanks to Karen Marshall, Jo Rittenhouse, Su Baker, and Timothy Richardson, M.D., for offering critical feedback regarding selected chapters.
- Friends who gave input and continued to love me even when the book came first, also Susan Perry, who taught me the importance of a good book proposal, and Tom, at Café Grande, who allowed me to sit and write for hours on end and for making the extraordinary lattes that kept me awake during this project.

- The many bodhisattvas who have touched my life, but especially the ones I was awake enough to embrace: Pat, Leni, Karla, and Joen. Words cannot adequately express my gratitude for having you as a part of my life.
- Milt, for your love, friendship, computer expertise, and unending support. And, of course, Alex and Miles, for your sloppy kisses and unconditional love.

Chapter One

Dissociation: An Overview

Have you ever headed for a particular destination and fallen so deep into thought that you missed your exit? I have. I used to be an educational consultant in western Kansas and would drive from school to school each day. If you have never been to Kansas, the images you may have conjured up from *The Wizard of Oz* or the various western novels you have read are probably close to the truth. I would grab a cup of coffee, get into my car, tune in the local radio station, and start driving to a particular school. One school was approximately twenty miles away from my house. The land was so flat and the scenery so desolate that the drive would become hypnotic and I would often miss my exit, not even realizing it until I started seeing signs for the next town up the road. You can probably think of similar situations in your own life. Maybe you have drifted so far during a lecture that the instructor was on to another topic by the time you mentally rejoined the group. Or maybe you are the type of person who can plop down on the sofa to watch your favorite movie and become so engrossed in the story that you do not even notice that your spouse is talking to you.

These normal experiences are simply brief periods of daydreaming and loss of awareness that psychologists refer to as dissociation. For the estimated one in a hundred people who are suffering from dissociative identity disorder (DID), however, lapses in awareness can be much more extreme and debilitating.[1] To understand a condition such as DID, the most extreme form of dissociation and the topic of this book, it helps to have a clear understanding of how dissociation works.

The brief hypnotic effect described above is just one aspect of dissociation. Another important aspect is dissociation's relationship to trauma. This type of dissociation is the type experienced by an individual with DID. It can be described as a disconnection. Some people say it is like being lost in a fog, whereas others state that the world around them seems very ethereal. When dissociated, people may feel disconnected from themselves, as if operating on autopilot. They may also feel disconnected from the world around them, as though there is an invisible force shield that prevents them from interacting with others. This disconnection can become so pervasive that the individual begins to distort time or, in extreme cases, actually loses time and recall of what happened during the dissociative period.

The roots of dissociation exemplify the mind/body connection, involving the brain, body, and emotions, and can be experienced in various ways. We all understand the experience of being so lost in our daydreams that we fail to notice the people around us. That type of experience falls into the category of normal dissociation. A trauma survivor, on the other hand, may not be able to remember entire blocks of time during the day. This type of dissociation falls into the category of *dysfunctional dissociation*. Dysfunctional dissociation is operative when

- an individual is not aware of or able to control her dissociative responses;
- these dissociative responses occur in inappropriate situations;
- the intensity and duration of the dissociation is disruptive to her life.[2]

We all use defenses when faced with overwhelming stress. These are what help to protect us emotionally. Dissociation is just one way people insulate themselves from pain. Even if the behavior falls into the category of dysfunctional dissociation, it does not mean that the person who is dissociating should feel shame. The dissociation actually served as a very adaptive and life-affirming defense at one point in time. The issue is that once the trauma is over and the threat no longer exists, the dissociation begins to interfere with life functioning, which is what makes it maladaptive in the present. This type of dissociation can then manifest in various psychological disorders, as illustrated in Table 1.1.

Posttraumatic stress disorder (PTSD) and *borderline personality disorder* (BPD) are also important to discussions related to trauma and dissociation. In the fourth edition of the *Diagnostic and Statistical Manual of Mental Disorders (DSM-IV)*, published by the American Psychiatric Association, PTSD is listed as an anxiety disorder and it is agreed that it is a response to trauma. In PTSD, traumatic events are reexperienced as intrusive thoughts, distressing dreams, flashbacks, and psychological or physical distress when the individual is reminded of the trauma. Persons with PTSD also tend to avoid things that remind them of the trauma they have experienced and they will use various responses, including dissociation, as a way of numbing themselves emotionally.[3]

Transient dissociation is one of the symptoms associated with BPD, and borderline individuals sometimes experience parts of the self as feeling separate. The ego states associated with BPD are not as compartmentalized as in DID, however, and loss of time is not associated with them. Many clinicians believe that BPD also develops as a result of severe neglect or other trauma experienced in early childhood.[4]

For the purposes of this book, however, the focus is on DID. PTSD is often a component of that diagnosis, and, in some cases, a DID client may be diagnosed with BPD as well. This material is being presented to explain the various aspects of dissociation. It is not meant to be used to self-diagnose. Yet, however a person experiences dissociation in

Table 1.1 Psychological Disorders Associated with Dissociation

Diagnosis	Definition
Amnesia	When a person has been traumatized or is experiencing extreme stress, she may find herself unable to recall important personal information, but the situation is much more serious than what you would expect with normal forgetfulness.
Fugue	An experience similar to amnesia except that the individual generally assumes a new life and has no recall for their own past.
Posttraumatic Stress Disorder (PTSD)	An anxiety disorder related to an individual's response to trauma. It often involves intrusive recall of the event, emotional numbing, increased arousal, or a combination of responses.
Depersonalization Disorder	A dissociative disorder in which an individual has recurrent experiences of feeling as if she is walking in a fog or a dream. Clients report that it seems as if they are observing themselves, yet they feel detached from their surroundings.
Borderline Personality Disorder (BPD)	A personality disorder involving a disturbance in identity and a pattern of impulsive behaviors and instability in relationship to self and others.
Dissociative Disorder Not Otherwise Specified (DDNOS)	Disorders in which dissociation is the primary symptom, but symptoms are not specific enough to meet the criteria for any of the other dissociative disorders. Examples include experiences similar to DID that either don't include two or more distinct personalities or do not include amnesia for important personal information.
Dissociative Identity Disorder (DID)	Formerly referred to as multiple personality disorder; described more fully later in this chapter.
Polyfragmented	A form of DID that often involves over one hundred DID personality states and is likely to be the result of cult abuse or some other form of extreme sadistic abuse that extends over a long period and often involves multiple perpetrators.
Somatization	Experiencing numerous physical complaints over several years beginning before the age of thirty.

(The information provided here is adapted from various sources, most notably the *Diagnostic and Statistical Manual of Mental Disorders*, 4th Ed., published by the American Psychiatric Association.)

regard to a particular diagnosis, one thing is clear: all dissociation results in an alteration in sense of awareness, whether it occurs in relationship to self, in relationship to memory, or in the way an individual interacts with the present environment. Someone reading this book may experience dissociation, or DID, or know someone who does.

TERMINOLOGY

If you know someone with DID, it helps to speak the language. Table 1.2 is a primer of need-to-know vocabulary.

The most important thing to remember when thinking about DID is that none of us has one totally integrated personality. DID is an extreme manifestation of what we all experience to a much lesser degree. For example, the typical person presents one side of herself at work, another when with friends, and yet another when at home with family. You may even refer to "parts" of your personality. Maybe you have found yourself doing so when faced with a decision. Your friends want you to go to a movie, and you cannot decide whether you want to do that or stick with your original plan of curling up in bed with a good book. You might find yourself saying, "Part of me wants to go to the movie and part of me wants to stay home." That thought does not mean that you are dissociative; it simply means that you are struggling with ambivalence. With BPD, the conflict might be experienced as more extreme, colored by thoughts about making the "right" decision. With DID, the experience goes to an even more extreme level in that distinct personality parts may hold the preferences of staying home versus going to a movie. In DID, the boundaries between personality parts are much more rigid and the personality parts themselves appear much more distinct.[5]

Table 1.2 DID Terms

Term	Definition
Alter	Short for alternate personality. In someone with DID, alters are dissociated parts of the self that represent memories, emotions, and ways of relating. They are able to function independently from each other and are also referred to as "parts" because they are parts of the individual's overall personality.
Co-consciousness	Awareness by one alter of the experience of other alters within the internal system of an individual with DID.
False memory	A term coined by the False Memory Syndrome Foundation to describe memories that they believe are not based on actual events. This concept is not yet proven by clinical research.
Flashback	Intrusive thoughts, feelings, or images associated with past trauma that suddenly enter into consciousness. Flashbacks often cause a person to feel as though he or she is reliving a traumatic event.
Fragment	A part of the self that lacks the emotional range or life history of an alter. Some fragments exist for very special purposes or roles and do not operate beyond the scope of these roles.

You might work with a manager every day and only see the work side of her personality. Then you get together for the company holiday party and she is telling jokes and acting like the life of the party. This behavior is normal. The interesting thing about DID is that the changes in a person's personality are sometimes no different than what occurred with the manager in this example. At other times, however, the changes may be so extreme that they are startling to those around that person.

Table 1.2 DID Terms, *continued*

Term	Definition
Fusion	Two alters coming together to form a single state.
Integration	The process of bringing dissociated material into consciousness.
Somatic flashback	Bodily sensations related to past trauma that has often been dissociated and not a part of the individual's conscious memory. Sometimes referred to as body memories.
Switching	Changing from one personality state to another. Sometimes accompanied by changes in physical appearance, vocal patterns, mood, or level of cognitive functioning. Many individuals report experiencing severe headaches in conjunction with switching.
System	A term describing all parts of the self in DID. A way of framing various parts as a whole as opposed to literal individual personalities.
Trigger	Something or someone that reminds a person of past trauma, whether or not the person is aware of the connection between the two. Triggers can include such things as people, odors, events, and objects.

DIAGNOSTIC CRITERIA

As mentioned earlier, when people think of DID, they generally think of Sybil. Sybil, played by Sally Field in the movie version, was diagnosed with multiple personalities resulting from severe child abuse. The book and the movie were quite graphic, and Sybil's various "parts" were distinct and easily recognized. In fact, the switching that occurred was often extreme. In reality, though, most individuals with DID do not present with such obvious switching. In addition to dissociation and the switching that often accompanies it, the major indicators of DID generally include such characteristics as inner voices, nightmares, panic attacks, depression, eating disorders, chemical dependency, loss of time, handwriting differences, differences in appearance, body memories, and severe headaches that are often associated with the switching behavior.[6] A client will not usually disclose the majority of these symptoms in the initial stages of treatment, however. That is why it is important for therapists to be trained to understand symptoms when they are presented so that they can be explored more fully. Although this topic is addressed in detail in chapter 3, let me share two possible situations that might occur in a therapy session.

First, if a client complained of hearing voices, it would be important for the therapist to explore the nature of the voices and how the person perceived them rather than assuming the client to be schizophrenic, which is what people usually think of when they hear someone talking about voices. Dissociators tend to hear inner voices that they perceive to be a part of themselves, which is very different from schizophrenia. Second, if a client appeared to be confused or preoccupied at a particular point in the session, it might be helpful for the therapist to ask what the client's internal experience had been and to find out whether she was aware of the conversation that had just taken place. If not, what may have just been experienced could be anything from mild dissociation to switching, yet these behaviors often go undetected.

Most of the characteristics associated with DID can be hidden from others fairly successfully. Granted, a DID friend or client might appear to be depressed, but how many other people have we all encountered who are depressed? Typically, someone with DID presents as moody or even a bit eccentric, but rarely as grossly abnormal.

The *Diagnostic and Statistical Manual of Mental Disorders*, 4th ed. (*DSM-IV*), states that the criteria given in Table 1.3 are currently necessary for a diagnosis of DID.

Table 1.3 Diagnostic Criteria for Dissociative Identity Disorder*

A. The presence of two or more distinct identities or personality states (each with its own relatively enduring pattern of perceiving, relating to, and thinking about the environment and self).

B. At least two of these identities or personality states recurrently take control of the person's behavior.

C. Inability to recall important personal information that is too extensive to be explained by ordinary forgetfulness.

D. The disturbance is not due to the direct physiological effects of a substance (e.g., blackouts or chaotic behavior during alcohol intoxication) or a general medical condition (e.g., complex partial seizures).

Note: In children, the symptoms are not attributable to imaginary playmates or fantasy play.

*Reprinted with permission from the *Diagnostic and Statistical Manual of Mental Disorders*, 4th ed. Copyright 1994 American Psychiatric Association.

My advice to clinicians is that until they have met an alter, it is not DID. They may suspect that someone has DID and their suspicions may prove to be correct, but each of the four criteria must be met to diagnose someone with DID. Until that time, a diagnosis such as dissociative disorder not otherwise specified (DDNOS) might be more appropriate. Chapter 3 discusses tools available to aid the therapist in diagnosis, but for now let us look at the way this disorder has been viewed throughout history.

HISTORY OF DISSOCIATION AND DID

From Eve to Sybil to Truddi Chase, the media has chronicled the lives of people with DID. Is this because of the controversy surrounding the diagnosis or because of the sensationalism associated with the individual stories? Whatever the motivation, one thing is sure: the public continues to gravitate toward the topic.

Nicole, however, is one who lives the story. She is a successful professional living in an urban area of the United States. For as long as she can remember, various "people" have held conversations in her head. She never thought to question this phenomenon. After all, if it was happening to her it must be commonplace. When the stress of everyday life finally became intolerable and the voices unrelenting, Nicole decided to seek the help of a therapist. One afternoon, during a routine therapy session, one of the "voices" decided to present herself in physical form. Nicole curled up on the couch and her face softened to such an extent that she actually began to look younger. Her words became whispers as she glanced shyly at the floor. The therapist, stunned by Nicole's dramatic change in appearance, asked a simple, yet poignant, question: "How old are you?" A childlike face on a woman's body responded, first by looking up, tentatively, as if confused about whether she should answer the question. Then, she looked at her hands and slowly counted her fingers until she reached the number 4. She held up her right hand, showing the therapist her four extended fingers, then quickly looked away. The therapist nodded with a kind and gentle smile that seemed to be communicating a sense of safety. Then, the therapist quietly spoke again. "Do you have a name?" "Rebecca," she answered. From that moment on, Nicole was not simply an adult woman addressing the issues that were creating anxiety in her life. She was a woman with a diagnosis of DID.

The first time that DID really hit the public eye was in 1957 with the Joanne Woodward film *The Three Faces of Eve*. The film was about Eve White, a depressed housewife who was also suffering from headaches and occasional blackouts. After finally seeing a psychiatrist, it was discovered that two other personalities existed within this woman. One was Eve Black, the wild, fun-loving antithesis of the original Eve. The other was Jane, the more insightful and stable aspect of the three. Because the film was based on a true story, it heightened public awareness of the disorder.

Sybil was a 1976 television movie starring Sally Field as a patient with MPD/DID and Joanne Woodward as the psychiatrist who treated her. Sybil became the modern version of Eve and is often the first association that people have when they hear the words MPD or DID. Despite the Hollywood blitz associated with this disorder, however, diagnosis appears to have begun much earlier, in the late 1800s with Pierre Janet, a French psychiatrist, and William James, a student of both philosophy and psychology. Then, in 1906, Morton Prince introduced the term *co-consciousness* to explain what takes place as a client becomes aware of the dissociative process and how it operates in her life. O'Regan further described dissociation as "an unconscious defense mechanism in which a group of mental activities split off from the main stream of consciousness and function as a separate unit."[7]

The purpose of dissociation is to take memory or emotion that is directly associated with a trauma and to encapsulate, or separate, it from the conscious self.

- Dissociation is a creative way of keeping the unacceptable out of sight.
- It is a way for the DID internal system to protect secrets and continually learn to adapt to the environment.
- It is a lifesaving defense.
- It allows an attachment to the abuser to be maintained.
- It allows strong, and often conflicting, emotions to be kept in separate compartments in the mind.

Why, though, does this topic continue to garner such attention within mental health circles? Training, of course, has a huge effect on all mental health professionals. If a therapist is trained to believe that DID does not exist, she is much more likely to interpret the condition as something a client is creating to manipulate the people around her or to simply misdiagnose it. Other professionals refuse to become a part of some of the extremism that was associated with the disorder in the past. DID was once considered to be very rare and bizarre. Many people, including mental health professionals, were fearful of it. The diagnosis carried an air of hysteria that often had more to do with the clinician's reaction to it than with that of the patient. Many clinicians feared being seen as extremists if they associated themselves with the treatment of the disorder.

In recent years, there has also been an increase in the number of lawsuits related to the purported misdiagnosis of DID by mental health professionals as well as an extreme backlash by groups such as the False Memory Syndrome Foundation in response to a more direct approach to the identification and treatment of past trauma in childhood. Some professionals become so ingrained in their own beliefs that they refuse to look at research or opinions that differ from their own. For some of these therapists, there is an excitement about treating a DID patient that appears to have more to do with experiencing the disorder than with treating the patient. For others, the opposite is true. These professionals have been so swayed by the sensationalism associated with DID that they are actually fearful of encountering someone with the disorder.

Anything that is controversial tends to divide people into theoretical "camps." Societal issues and beliefs affect the therapeutic community in much the same ways that the general population is affected. Because DID is so often associated with sexual abuse, it falls under the "do not talk rule" that is prominent in dysfunctional families and, at times, in entire societies. In the matter of child abuse, it appears that entire countries have gone through periods of mass denial. People prefer to believe that bad things do not happen in their own neighborhoods. Yet despite the political underpinnings, most clinicians are simply interested in helping the people who come to them. So, if clients look for a therapist who is experienced in treating DID or, at the very least, willing to learn, they cannot go too far astray.

Basic misunderstandings about DID encountered in the therapeutic community include the following:

- The expectation that all clients with DID will present in a Sybil-like manner, with obvious switching and extreme changes in personality.
- That therapists create DID in their clients.
- That DID clients have very little control over their internal systems and can be expected to stay in the mental health system indefinitely.
- That alter personalities, especially child alters, are simply regressive states associated with anxiety or that switching represents a psychotic episode.

Anyone who experiences dissociation on a regular basis knows better, however. DID is not only disruptive to everyday life but is also confusing and, at times, frightening. Allow me to paint a picture of what an experience with dissociation might be like.

The typical DID client talks about hearing voices in her head since childhood. Initially, she assumes that such voices are common to everyone. As she continues to grow, however, life becomes more unmanageable. The voices may comment on her behavior or may even appear to be controlling her. In the 1960s, comedian Flip Wilson popularized a character by the name of Geraldine who always explained her behavior away by quipping, "The devil made me do it." The DID client, however, actually does feel that someone else is making her behave in ways outside her norm, causing behaviors that may seem so out of character that she feels at times as if she is another person.

Then there are the constant accusations from others, such as, "You said you'd call me last night. Don't you remember?" The reality is that she may not remember. Others, though, seem so sure of what she said that she begins to doubt herself. If she does deny what the other person is saying, it is assumed that she is joking or is lying.

CURRENT THINKING

As more and more research is being done regarding the effects of trauma, we are learning about the brain's influence during and after traumatic events and how memory is affected. Because a trauma is an experience that is extremely distressing and generally is met with fear and feelings of powerlessness, dissociation is a common response. It allows persons experiencing the trauma to change their consciousness in a way that permits them to distance or disconnect from the full impact of what is happening. That distancing can take place in terms of memory, emotion, the actual physical experience, or, in more extreme cases, sense of identity. When under threat, the brain defaults to the biology of survival.[8] Therefore, dissociation can be thought of as both a neurobiological response to threat and a psychological defense at work to protect one from an overwhelming experience.

What makes the defense of dissociation become a diagnosis of dissociation is the severity and way it operates. Think again of dissociation and the very ordinary ways that most of us dissociate, as in the case of highway hypnosis. Then take things a step further, to the individual who regularly uses dissociation as a defense. This person "numbs out" when faced with overwhelming stress. As long as the numbing does not happen too often or become too severe, it serves as a way for the person to separate from stress that feels too difficult to handle. Once the dissociation becomes frequent enough or severe enough to interfere with life functioning, however, the person is likely to seek help and find an actual diagnosis.

Dissociation is a common symptom experienced by people suffering from PTSD. When reminded of past trauma, a Vietnam veteran might dissociate to keep from being flooded with memories. When dissociation is more pervasive, however, as is the case with DID, it becomes a typical part of a person's daily coping style, which, of course, can become extremely problematic for the person experiencing it.

One problem is that a person may become so adept at using dissociation that conscious memories of a traumatic event are tucked away only to emerge at a later time. One of the most common ways that these memories begin to resurface is through experiences referred to as flashbacks. During a flashback, it may feel as if an experience is being relived. Another common occurrence is nightmares that feel very real and may even be difficult to distinguish from the waking world. These intrusive images often prompt people to seek treatment.

Another issue related to memory is that its content can change over time and circumstances. There are different forms of memory. Explicit memory is what we usually think of when we talk about memory. It is the kind of memory we use for recalling facts and events or any information from the past that is consciously available. Implicit memory, however, differs in form. It is the type of experience in which you know something but do not explicitly remember how you know, as with behaviors and attitudes that have simply become "a part of you." Because implicit memory is thought to be involved in the processing of strong emotions, it is understandable why some traumatic memory might be experienced primarily as emotion or physical sensation rather than as concrete vocabulary.

Memory naturally changes over time as we continue to learn and grow. As we make sense of our lives, we fill in the blanks of our memories and create an ever-changing narrative of who we are in the midst of our life experiences. It appears, however, that traumatic memory does not change significantly over time, which is one reason flashbacks and unexplainable bodily sensations can create such a sense of panic as they begin to emerge.[9]

UNDERSTANDING THE PARTS OF THE SELF

To understand DID fully, it is important to understand how different parts function. Dissociators often refer to these parts as alters. There are many similarities regarding the roles of alters, although each internal system will function according to a person's unique experience and personality. Therapists are more likely to operate from a framework that defines alters as ego states, or parts of the self, so as to reinforce that they are actually various aspects of one self. An ego state may form based on a group of emotions or experiences. Although separate, and able to act more or less independently in the world, they are still a part of a whole person who is fragmented and compartmentalized.[10]

Carla's system is one example of how alters might function. She has a four-year-old child part who experienced the initial trauma. This child's main function is to carry the memory of the trauma, a bizarre ritual in which she was sexually abused. She also carries the fear that was experienced during the ritual, a fear so intense that Carla has managed to keep it out of her own consciousness.

There are other child alters in Carla's system, as well. One is a ten-year-old-boy named Carl who also carries memories of past abuse as well as the anger that was needed to survive. Carl has also taken on the role of protecting the girls in the system and often emerges if he thinks any of the younger parts are feeling frightened.

Carla also plays host to two teenagers. One is Carly, age sixteen, who was raped while in a dissociated state and unable to defend herself. Like Carl, Carly holds the emotion of anger and often "comes out" in situations where Carla is angry, but feels unable to express herself. The problem is, the anger is usually expressed in the way you might expect any sixteen-year-old to express it. So when thirty-five-year-old Carla switches and begins to express her anger in a defiant and rebellious manner, the people around her are left feeling perplexed by the sudden change in mood and attitude.

Internal parts can be thought to be a result of the dissociative process and as containing specific memories, experiences, emotions, or styles of functioning. Initially, parts are so compartmentalized that the dissociator may not be aware of them. Even as awareness increases, however, the parts continue to be experienced as separate identities, even though they are actually parts of the person's mind. They tend to operate as highly distinct and recognizable to others who get to know the individual's internal system well. To the rest of the world, though, they may appear only as shifts in mood that are sometimes extreme or do not seem appropriate to the situation. Individuals with DID unconsciously form these parts. Yet it is interesting to note that DID clients often share similarities in the way that they function internally and may even refer to the parts with labels that describe their functions, such as host, child alters, persecutors, and protectors. These parts are created to function in specific ways. The host can be thought of as the part having control of the body the greatest percentage of time. Often this is the part who comes for therapy. The presenting problem tends to be anxiety or depression, and the individual may or may not suspect that she has DID. The child parts will often hold the memories of the trauma or the corresponding emotions. They may represent different ages when the trauma was significant and even present as a child that age in terms of speech or physical appearance. They may or may not be able to talk, read, or write. Sometimes they grow chronologically and other times they do not, but it is very typical for a system to have parts that exhibit age-appropriate behaviors normally associated with childhood or adolescence. Another aspect of child parts, however, is that they may be based on childhood fantasy or the "idealized child," in which case they may not hold memories of the trauma but instead have formed an identity based on what they believed or wanted to believe about themselves and their families. One example of an idealized child is the "good little girl" who behaves in the way that she believes is expected, regardless of whether or not this belief is based on fact. Another is the child from the "perfect" family who in turn must be the "perfect" child. Other idealized states may be based on fairy tales or heroines from childhood storybooks or movies.

Some ego states represent *introjects* (characteristics of the abuser that become internalized by the victim) of the abusers. An "abuser" ego state may develop from the person internalizing aspects of an actual abuser or in response to the abuser. These parts can be frustrating to therapists because they seem to be undermining treatment at times. Functionally, these parts may be trying to protect the individual from perceived danger from the outside world, but if they are operating with a distorted view of reality, they often "protect" in ways that do not make sense to those on the outside. These parts may also try to protect the individual from the toxic shame that causes them to believe that they are defective in comparison with others. They may appear grandiose at times or attacking, as a means of insulating the DID individual from the outside world. Some people with DID report having parts that inflict harm to the body. They may emerge when the individual feels threatened or may harm the body to silence the person, thus keeping secrets from being exposed.

> Sandy was raised in a family that was involved in multigenerational cult activity. Although she is aware of the cult abuse, she continues to dissociate aspects of the abuse that she feels unable to handle emotionally. One of her alters is an imposing male figure that emerges when Sandy tries to talk about specific aspects of the abuse. What Sandy has learned from internal communication with her system is that this nameless, faceless figure was created by the cult to keep her from telling anyone what was happening. In early adulthood, when Sandy began to have memories of the abuse, this alter began threatening her. She would wake up from dissociative states with coffee and cigarette burns on her arms and notes that threatened her to "keep the secrets to yourself."

In essence, all parts can be thought of as being protectors, with some being more functional and reality based than others. Some may function to soothe younger parts. Others may provide valuable information and insight to the client and therapist and are often the most aware of how the system functions overall. Some clients even experience these parts as spiritual entities that are separate from themselves. However they present, ego states that are perceived as protectors are vital in helping the client to regain a sense of empowerment.

There may be one or several parts functioning in a particular role. Typically, the most splitting occurs in situations where the trauma is severe and long lasting. In systems where extreme splitting occurs, clients may report a host of personality fragments created to do specific tasks, such as cooking, cleaning the house, or going to school.

Once the task is performed, the fragment becomes inactive. It is important for nondissociators to notice that they probably operate differently according to the task at hand as well; it is simply a matter of degree. We all have the ability to compartmentalize when under stress. That is what allows therapists, for example, to continue to see clients when they are also experiencing stress in their own lives. When therapists see clients, they know that they will be focusing on one person for one hour. If therapists are particularly stressed about a personal issue, they know that they must put it away until they either have a break in the day or have left the office and gone home. That is healthy adaptation. Even though DID creates more extreme compartmentalizing, it also helps the individual to adapt and balance the various responsibilities in a given day.

If you think about the different parts of your own personality, it will help you, in a small way, to envision what life is like for a dissociator. Think about your professional persona, your role as a spouse, your parental role, and the side of your personality that is most prevalent when with various friends. Now imagine magnifying those roles without allowing them to intersect at all, and you will have a small taste of what it is like to live with DID.

THE BRAIN AND DISSOCIATION

If dissociation is initially helpful when dealing with trauma yet very unhelpful once the danger has passed, why do people continue the process? The answer lies in part with a small primitive area of the brain called the *amygdala*, which is thought to assess and respond to potential threats before conscious awareness even occurs.

One way of thinking about trauma is to imagine it being processed through the thalamus on its journey to the prefrontal cortex, where the traumatized individual is able to make sense of the experience. On its journey to the frontal cortex, the information is filed in the appropriate file folder (or context) to be brought out later, if necessary. If the information is not adequately processed, however, the cortex begins to operate like a sentry, working hard to guard the limbic system and to keep the traumatic material at bay. Unfortunately, the cortex does not work well when someone is asleep, overly tired, drinking, or especially when experiencing any form of PTSD. Trauma researcher Bessel van der Kolk and colleagues hypothesize that PTSD occurs in part when the amygdala overfunctions and the hippocampus underfunctions.[11] In other words, the trauma hits like a hurricane, the amygdala cannot withstand the force, the hippocampus shuts down in fear, the information is not put into the appropriate file folders, and the traumatic experience floods the central nervous system.

The limbic system of the brain (made up in part by the amygdala, hippocampus, thalamus, and hypothalamus) is primitive and reactive in the way it interprets incoming information. Because language is not a part of the limbic system's repertoire, that information is interpreted as images and sensations. We make meaning in the frontal lobe of the brain where feelings and thoughts join together to create a unified story about our experiences.[12]

In reality, the processing of trauma is much more complex than this explanation and, naturally, DID develops over a course of events, not just a single episode. What we call memory, be it traumatic or not, is the interpretation and integration of many life experiences coming together to form a single narrative, referred to as *semantic memory*.

More and more research is being done on the way the brain processes trauma, which will be key to furthering our understanding and ability to treat trauma survivors successfully. Until then, we do the best we can. DID is a prime example of how survivors do just that. It truly is a lifesaving response to overwhelming life experiences.

THE EFFECTS OF TRAUMA

The effects of dissociation are far-reaching and change in form and intensity depending on an individual's own experience at the time. If the issue is one of self-regulation, which is a common characteristic of borderline personality disorder, a person might find that it is difficult to keep emotions at a level that feels tolerable. Anger seems to be an especially difficult emotion to manage, probably because of the amount of anger that has had to be repressed over the years as a means of survival. Clients often say that they are fearful of expressing anger lest they rage out of control. Of course, survivors of abuse have often seen just that in their perpetrators. They are unable to recognize that anger does not have to equal rage and that not all anger has to be acted on. This issue is one that leads to a preoccupation with self-harm. Harmful behaviors directed at one's self can be a way of expressing the anger that has been carried for so long. It is also a way of feeling. If the dissociation is effective enough to create a pervasive "numbing out," self-harm is a way for people to remind themselves that they are alive.

The most extreme form of self-harm is suicide, which provides a permanent means of escape. "I am going to kill myself" can become a kind of mantra for someone who lives with intense pain. Although the conscious desire may be to live, such a person can hold on to suicide as an option in case life becomes too intolerable. Sometimes when a person believes she has a way out, she feels less trapped and better equipped to face life. I certainly do not advocate suicide as a viable option, but I can understand it. Through reading this book and partnering with a good therapist, someone who is dissociative can learn healthier alternatives for dealing with her pain.

Alteration in consciousness is another response to trauma that dissociators experience, and as discussed earlier, it can present as amnesia, depersonalization, or dissociation. A third response is *somatization*: emotional pain that is translated into physical pain. This response is not about it being "all in your head." It is about the very real experience of body/mind being one. Because it is impossible to operate in one without the other, it is natural to assume that what happens to someone emotionally will be expressed in the body as well. It is one way of giving witness to the pain she has endured.

Identity issues affect the person with DID and also the way she views life in many ways. People with DID often blame themselves for what was done to them. Intellectually, they are quick to put the blame where it belongs. "Of course I am not responsible for my father molesting me. I was only seven years old." At a deeper level, however, they do feel responsibility and an intense amount of shame. They might feel different from other people and find that this feeling carries over into relationships with others. Often, persons who have been abused have difficulty trusting others even when all the evidence points to the contrary. As a result, they may find that they continue to play out the victim and perpetrator roles in their current relationships.

Kate was molested by her father, and the abuse lasted from the age of five to age twelve. Her father would come into her room at night and fondle her, telling her that he loved her and that she was special to him. Kate loved her father, too, but felt fearful whenever he would come into her room at night. As with most perpetrators, he told her that his actions were a secret and that no one could ever know. He also told Kate that her mother would be very angry with her if she knew what was happening and that the two of them would probably never be allowed to see each other again. Kate did what most victims do. She kept the secret.

Now, as an adult, Kate has difficulty trusting others. When people are nice to her, she looks for ulterior motives. She allows people to take advantage of her, especially people in authority. Her coworkers never have to worry about whether a job will get done because Kate will shoulder the bulk of the responsibility. Yet, despite her victim role, Kate's anger is often unleashed on others. She may get the job done, but her biting remarks directed at others in the office create a tension that does not easily disappear. It all began because a father molested his little girl.

When a person is traumatized in her formative years, the sense of self is unable to fully develop. Therapy is about constructing that self so that an individual can operate more effectively in the world, but from a stronger internal base. Still, if the DID developed as a result of abuse, part of a discussion of relationships, as in the case of Kate, must include the perpetrator. The perpetrator may have been an individual, as in incest, or a system, as in cult abuse. Whichever the case, a person has to come to terms eventually with how she views the perpetrator(s). This view will probably change as she goes through the course of therapy, and she is bound to experience some ambivalence along the way. At times, she will probably identify with the perpetrator and may even idealize him. At other times she may experience rage and a preoccupation to "get even." Often, victims will adopt some of the distorted thinking of the perpetrator and act as if such thinking is true. In the case of DID, certain ego states may even represent introjects of the perpetrator, which serve to keep the abuse going in the form of self-abuse or abuse toward others.

Therapy does not end when parts reach a final fusion or integration into one self. Survivors are constantly reinterpreting the trauma and creating new ways of understanding their stories. Part of therapy has to do with learning to live life as an integrated being who takes the despair and hopelessness of the past trauma and learns to transform them in much the same way that Rumplestiltskin spun straw into gold. Before the trauma, the person carried certain beliefs about life. As a result of the trauma, those beliefs were altered. Now the person's job is to refashion beliefs about self and the world. This part of the grieving process is a major identifier of the quest for health. Trauma alters a person's sense of reality. Therapy helps create a new reality.

In chapter 2 we begin to look at the personal "reality" behind the development of DID and how an adaptive response to trauma can eventually become maladaptive as well.

Chapter Two

Creative Coping or Dysfunction? You Be the Judge

Cassie is a student at a state university. She carries a full class load, maintains a 3.8 grade point average, and also works part-time to help with college expenses. Yet, in the midst of her busy schedule, Cassie experiences losses of time ranging from minutes to entire days and is often surprised to find threatening notes to herself admonishing her to "keep it together or pay the price." She is frightened and struggling to keep her life on an even keel, but she finds it more and more difficult to do so. She wants to seek the help of a therapist, but she fears that she will be labeled "crazy" and branded for the rest of her life.

Even in today's "enlightened" society, the stigma of mental illness remains. It is frightening to think about carrying such a label, and much of that fear is about wondering what the label means. If I am mentally ill, does that mean I'll be suicidal? Does it mean I'll hear voices? Will they lock me up and throw away the key? Worse yet, can people see the label simply by looking at me?

DEVELOPMENT OF DID

There are various types of mental disorders. Some, such as schizophrenia or bipolar disorder, are thought to be biologically based and are treated in part by medications that aid in the management of symptoms. Other disorders have more to do with difficulties in daily living and can be related to trauma, grief and loss, situational stressors, internal conflict, or attachment issues resulting from neglect or extremely inconsistent parenting styles. Over time, professionals have debated the classification, and even the existence, of DID. It is difficult to prove its existence biologically, so the dilemma is created. Is it mental illness or a style of functioning? What is known about DID is that it is a developmental disorder.[1] If an individual is traumatized in early childhood and the experience is so overwhelming that he is unable to process it, the child may dissociate to survive. DID results when the dissociation becomes severe enough to allow the child to compartmentalize parts of himself from consciousness and experience them as separate from the core self. We can all identify with mild dissociation because we do it on a regular basis; we simply call it daydreaming or spacing out. More severe dissociation, however, looks different.

Tim is five years old. Mom stays at home to raise him, and Dad has a sales job that sends him out on the road frequently. Dad also drinks abusively. Tim's world is pretty standard. He goes to school, plays with neighborhood children, and loves having his mother read to him before bed each night. On those nights when Dad comes in drunk and angry, though, anything that's close to normal quickly disappears. Spilled milk will result in yelling and name calling. If Mom dares to intervene, the result is usually physical abuse. Tim is only five, yet he's facing the rage of a man in his late thirties. He does not have any physical defenses, but he can make himself "go away." While Dad yells, Tim sits quietly. Then, when the fear becomes too much to handle, he projects himself into a corner of the room and another little boy, Matthew, takes the father's abuse. Later, when it begins to feel safe again, Tim rejoins his body.

Tim does not consciously go through these motions, and he certainly does not refer to it as dissociation, but he is adapting to a frightening and potentially dangerous situation through his behavior. For a child to develop the capacity to cope in this manner seems nothing less than miraculous.

The human brain is built to process trauma, but it is not meant to have to process severe trauma on an ongoing basis. So, when the brain becomes overwhelmed with traumatic stimuli, several things begin to happen. In some cases, some of the stimuli simply make the brain act as though it is stuck, much like a videotape that has become worn. In Tim's situation, that broken tape might replay a horrifying scene of his father beating his mother as he sits by helplessly. The scene may wake him up at night or intrude into his thoughts during the day, making it difficult to concentrate on schoolwork or normal play.

MENTAL DISORDERS AND ADAPTIVE FUNCTIONING

What are the differences between mental disorders and adaptive functioning? For that matter, do they need to be mutually exclusive? DID is classified as a diagnosable mental disorder in the *Diagnostic and Statistical Manual of Mental Disorders (DSM-IV)*. When something is diagnosable according to *DSM-IV* standards, it means that a pattern of behavior or other criteria are present the majority of the time for the diagnosis being considered. Some argue that DID should not be listed in the manual and that doing so creates even more of a stigma for those who experience the disorder. Yet DID is diagnosable because there are symptoms present that interfere with daily functioning. A neurobiological component involved with the processing of trauma is included as well. It is how the brain is involved, however, that makes the classification of DID so controversial.

DID is similar to PTSD in the way that brain functioning is involved. It is a result of severe trauma, and the resulting hyperarousal is connected to the amygdala in the same way that PTSD is. The main difference between the two disorders is that individuals with DID unconsciously compartmentalize parts of their minds and then push those parts outside of their consciousness, which is somewhat different from the emotional numbing that occurs with PTSD. Typically, what sets internal parts into motion is either emotion that has been cut off from consciousness or hyperarousal in the brain that causes the person with DID to react as though she is faced with extreme danger even when she is not. When this happens on a consistent basis, it will interfere with normal functioning.

Karen is an art instructor. She is successful in her work, and her students adore her. There are days, however, when she is unable to be fully present with her students due to severe headaches that no amount of medication will take away. She does not know why the headaches plague her, and no medical reason has been found. All she can pinpoint is that the internal pressure is enormous, and when the headaches hit she begins to feel younger and more vulnerable. She is still able to teach, but she is not able to connect with her students in her usual relaxed manner. It is as if she is operating from a vacuum. She goes through the motions, yet she does not actually feel as if she is there. Once the day is over, she goes home, as if in a trance, and goes to bed. Sometimes she wakes up feeling perfectly normal again. More often than not, however, she experiences nightmares or wakes up in the night feeling as if someone is in the room. She knows she is safe, yet everything she is *experiencing* internally says otherwise. On some days, the intensity of the headaches combined with lack of sleep become too much so she calls in sick just to get some sleep and, she hopes, gain some perspective.

Is mental illness shown here? Physical symptoms are experienced, daily living is disrupted, and emotions are affected. Yet the tendency to describe situations such as this one as mental illness may have more to do with the way they manifest themselves. When we see an individual's emotions changing, behavior typically changes as well. Often, thinking becomes distorted, which can be frightening to those people close by. In Karen's case, a diagnosis of DID has not been made yet because the disruption to her life has not been severe enough. Most people with DID can point to examples much like Karen's in their own lives that signaled something was not quite right. It is not unusual for different parts to manifest symptoms of anxiety, depression, or other disorders. When those disorders are appearing in sync with the switching of alters, the individual's changes in mood and behavior can be quite distressing to everyone involved. It is easy to see why a person with DID would be labeled as mentally ill by those closest to him or by mental health professionals unfamiliar with the diagnosis. Yet to peers and casual friends, the behavior of someone with DID tends to be more mystifying than alarming.

When a dissociator is triggered by some sort of external stimuli, an internal response that is associated with past trauma is created. Others might view the resulting behavior as an overreaction or a shutting down that does not quite fit the situation, but if the dissociator's internal system is highly functional, the more overt symptoms may remain hidden. So, if DID is a response to past trauma, which is external, how can it be considered a mental illness? Many people with DID balk at the use of the term *disorder*. When every ounce of your being comes together to fight for survival, having it termed a disorder can feel discounting, to say the least. Because the traditional concept of mental illness continues to carry a negative stigma with the expectation of long-term treatment and little progress, many prefer to think in terms of creating positive movement rather than perpetuating a negative stereotype. Looking for client strengths is the first step in that direction. So, if we were to start by making a case for adaptive functioning, where might it lead us?

ADAPTIVE FUNCTIONING

Let's start by defining adaptive functioning. In psychological terms, adaptation is seen as an attempt to reach a state of equilibrium in the face of pressure originating from both internal and external stressors. Adaptation has been a part of humanity since the beginning of humankind. If I need to walk on two legs to survive, I learn to walk on two legs. If I need fire and tools to survive, I develop tools and learn how to use fire in ways that will benefit me. This behavior is adaptation. Throughout our lives, we learn to adapt. A child learns to crawl and then learns to walk. She moves from cooing, to babbling, to forming words, phrases, and eventually complete sentences. We can only guess how much of such adaptation is inborn and how much is learned, but we do know that the more able a person is to adapt, the more successful she will be. In centuries past, adapting meant survival, literally. Today, however, adapting often takes on a more emotional significance as well. The people who are most successful in modern society tend to be those who are able to recognize emotional states in self and others, manage their own emotions, and adapt when situations and emotions are not what they would like them to be.

In the case of DID, normal emotional states are often experienced as being very extreme. Because those reactions were probably developed in response to childhood trauma, that would make sense. A child, whose brain is still developing and who is faced with painful, even life-threatening experiences that he is not yet equipped to handle, will be overwhelmed. To split off that terror from consciousness is extremely adaptive and means emotional and, possibly, physical survival. If Billy's father is beating him with a belt and Billy is able to imagine that the abuse is happening to another little boy as opposed to himself, that is adaptive functioning for a child.

You can think of adaptive functioning as survival. Granted, not all survival is related to life-threatening issues, but getting daily needs met is a means of survival nonetheless. Psychologist Abraham Maslow developed a hierarchy that brilliantly illustrates our survival instincts, ranging from our needs for food, water, and shelter at the bottom of the hierarchy all the way up to self-actualization at the top. The importance of this hierarchy is Maslow's insight into the importance of meeting basic needs before moving onto higher-level needs. Not only is it important, but it is a prerequisite.[2] Imagine a young woman in her early twenties who experiences terrifying flashbacks on a daily basis, yet who is working on completing a college degree. Can it be done? The answer is probably, but at what cost? Her goal of earning a degree will be much more realistic if she attends to managing her emotions and the intrusive thoughts related to them. Until then, she is expending incredible energy in an attempt to concentrate on schoolwork while keeping inner distractions at bay. To simply stop and learn the necessary skills for managing the flashbacks before turning back to her schoolwork will save this woman both emotional and physical energy, not to mention money. Now imagine what life would be like for this woman if she were homeless. Until her basic needs of food, water, and shelter are met, completing school is not even an option.

Although basic survival needs come first, it appears that PTSD is more likely to develop in individuals who lack the necessary social support for processing the trauma. Consequently, they end up feeling completely overwhelmed by the emotional or physical results of their experience and at a loss as to how to manage the situation. It appears that lack of social support, coupled with a real or perceived lack of resources, is a strong indicator that someone will develop PTSD following a trauma, with dissociation at the time of the trauma being the biggest predictor of all.[3] Yet that they survive at all is part of the adaptive process. Their own resiliency is at work even if they cannot yet recognize it. If adaptive functioning can be thought of as resiliency and the survival instinct at work, how does it play out for individuals with DID?

Shari was five years old when she was raped by a group of teenage boys in the neighborhood. She was terrified and wanted to cry out for her parents to help her, but the boys taunted her by screaming, "Crybaby," "We'll tell your daddy how bad you are and you'll be punished," and "If you tell anybody about it, we'll sneak into your house at night and kill you." Although only five, Shari was able to quickly make a judgment about what to do. She shut her mouth and kept the screams inside herself. Then, as each of the three boys climbed on top of her, she went deeper inside of herself to avoid the pain. With each step inward, another part of herself stepped forward to experience the emotional and physical pain of the rapes. She was alone. Utterly alone. So she created internal parts to shield herself from the terror. Without that level of survival at work in her mind and body, Shari could easily have died.

For Mike it was a little different. The abuse was almost a daily experience. If Dad was sober or absent for some reason, Mike was granted a reprieve, but it didn't happen often. Mike's life went something like this: get up, eat breakfast, and go to school. He loved school because it offered a sense of safety. He also got validation there. Mike was an A and B student and naturally gifted intellectually. Teachers loved him. He was cooperative and threw himself into his work. School gave him a sense of mastery and control over life. At 3 o'clock each afternoon, though, the school day came to an end. Sometimes Mike would hang around the classroom to see if he could help the teacher in any way, other days he would play with friends, but most days he would wander the streets between school and home, delaying what he knew would await him at home. He knew he had to be there by supper or the punishment would be severe. So he always managed to make it before his father's arrival at 6 o'clock. Then, like his other siblings, he would go to the table and wait quietly to see what Dad's mood for the evening was going to be. If Dad was happy, everyone would breathe a quiet sigh of relief, especially Mike, the usual target of Dad's abuse. If Dad was angry or, worse yet, drunk and angry, however, there was no escaping his wrath.

Mike had become so adept at sensing his father's moods that he had developed an internal system that operated like clockwork. Mike sat down at the supper table and watched his father. If he was in a good mood, Mickey would come forward to joke with Dad and keep him feeling good. If Dad were in an angry mood, Michael would come out because he was much better at sparring verbally with Dad without losing his own temper and making things worse. And if Dad were both angry and drunk, the typical combination preceding physical abuse, Michael would stand at his post until the first swing. Then he would quickly change places with James, the tough teen who fought back. Not only was this adaptive on Mike's part, but it all occurred outside of his own consciousness.

BRAIN MATURATION AND EMOTIONAL MANAGEMENT

One of the main culprits in the adaptive functioning arena is emotion run amok. Brain maturity allows us to have feelings. So, generally speaking, when an adult experiences a feeling such as sadness, he knows that the feeling will eventually pass. Children, though, are their feelings. It is much more difficult for a child to differentiate between a feeling of sadness and the reality that he is separate from that feeling. We observe this in children all the time. When disappointments hit, especially in relationships, many children react as if it is the end of the world. Despite what some parents may think, this reaction is not simply a case of melodrama; it is really the reflection of a still-developing brain. Yet it is also related to learning and the developmental stages we pass through on the way to adulthood.

Much of what is experienced emotionally in childhood, in terms of process, is replayed in the adult with DID. The individual feels something negative, and, typically, the feeling is interpreted as being dangerous and overwhelming. For example, if you are in bed at 11 o'clock at night and the dog starts to bark, you might feel fear. At that point, you will make a quick decision either to check out the noise or to tell yourself it is probably nothing and go back to sleep. If you have DID and are put in the same situation, you are much more likely to go from fear to panic before being able to assess whether there is any real danger. The end result is an adult who feels very vulnerable and unable to manage her feelings.

There are many questions to be answered regarding this phenomenon if DID is to be understood and dealt with effectively. First, if DID is related to brain maturation, why doesn't the individual grow out of it? Second, how does it relate to the discussion of adaptive functioning? And, most important, how can it be dealt with?

This issue of emotion management has to do with how memory is formed. Early memories are stored as imprints, rather than narrative, because speech is not yet developed. In addition, the central nervous system is continuing to develop, even after birth. Until the temporal and frontal lobes are fully developed, it is impossible to store memory in narrative form. Thus, in early childhood, from infancy to approximately age three, feelings are experienced as a part of the self.[4] Young children do not think in terms of a separate self who is interacting with the mother or feeling fear. Instead, they experience themselves as part of everyone and everything that is happening in their worlds.

Sometimes, after watching science fiction movies, I fantasize about what it would be like to enter another time dimension or universe. Imagine how difficult it would be to separate yourself from your experience if you were the only human being in a parallel universe. If you sit in the safety of your own home and think about it, that kind of experience might seem kind of exciting. If you were actually catapulted into another galaxy and were totally alone, though, I do not think the feelings would all be positive ones. In fact, you just might begin to lose a bit of your sense of self (or you might begin to lose a lot of your sense of self!).

I certainly do not remember what it was like to be an infant, but I wonder if it is not somewhat like being transported to another planet. You leave the warmth and security of the womb and enter a world of bright lights and cold probing instruments amidst a sea of unrecognizable faces and voices. The good thing is that most babies are welcomed into this world with loving and nurturing parents. As they develop, memory begins with feeling that is translated into different somatic sensations; thus, the hungry cry, the sleepy cry, and the wet diaper cry. Nurturing parents quickly respond to those cries. As the child grows, he reaches a stage of development where he gradually begins to realize that he is a separate being: Mommy is one person, Daddy is another, and I am another. With the development of language, the child then learns to create stories to explain the various feelings that come and go.

DEVELOPMENTAL ISSUES

In DID, these younger parts might be thought of as developmental stages that are encapsulated and stored inside the brain. This thinking helps explain why a thirty-four-year-old man can go to the office and operate effectively, but become a frightened five-year-old if he is alone at night during a thunderstorm. The feelings related to the storm may trigger memories of something he experienced as a five-year-old, and conscious attention turns to that part of himself. If the memory is stored in his body as a somatic or physical sensation, this man will feel fear and will react accordingly, but if he is reacting from a five-year-old's perspective, he is also likely to forget that he is an adult who is separate from the feelings of fear that he is currently experiencing. Similar situations are played out again and again in the lives of individuals with DID.

So, in the case of DID, the issue is not entirely one of brain maturation. It is mainly about connecting with those parts of the self that are younger and integrating them into the larger aspect of self. Yes, technically the dissociator is dealing with issues related to the brain's ability to process information and to store that information into memory, but the dissociator is also introducing the concept of dissociation into an already fragmented picture. Think of this as a giant jigsaw puzzle of a person's life. Some pieces represent the conscious adult life that she is living now. Others represent past memories, some of which are remembered clearly and others that are experienced more like a walk in the fog. This person might remember aspects of the experience, but it will be incomplete and not always believable to her conscious mind. Even so, the fog limits the mind's eye in its ability to see. Other pieces of the puzzle appear as somatic sensations that represent memory that has been repressed, what some refer to as "body memories." A somatic flashback may be played out as a stomachache that begins when a woman is watching television and sees an unexpected molestation occur in the movie she is watching. This flashback is not related to consciousness, but to the memory of a past experience that has been stored in her body at a cellular level.

DEVELOPMENTAL STAGES OF CHILDHOOD

Various developmental theories in the fields of psychology and education reflect and agree on one thing: the path from infancy to adulthood provides mile markers along the way that allow us to gauge our distance on the road to maturity. Child development is not the primary focus of this book, but it does bear mentioning because of its relationship to the way internal parts operate in DID.

Piaget

Psychologist Jean Piaget paved the way for research into child development. He talked about the different ways in which children and adults approach thinking. One difference lies in the area of *concrete* versus *formal operations*. Children in the concrete realm focus on the relationship between objects. In this stage, if a child is shown two identical glasses containing the same amounts of water, he will judge them to be equal. If water is poured from one of the glasses into a narrower container, however, creating a higher level, the child will say that the container with the higher level contains more water. The development of formal thinking allows us to think abstractly, to use logical reasoning, and to hypothesize and use deductive reasoning, which are all higher-level functions; but an individual does not operate formally without first going through the concrete. We build on previously learned skills through functions that Piaget refers to as assimilation, accommodation, and equilibration. *Assimilation* has to do with incorporating new pieces of information into our thinking, *accommodation* refers to how we make room for the new information, and *equilibration* describes the way we balance the old beliefs with the new information.

Suppose that a child held a firm belief that the earth is flat, based on his perception of the world. Then he learns from his teacher that the world is, in fact, round. He decides to do a bit of research and finds information that supports what the teacher is saying. From the moment the child hears that the world is round, he begins the process of assimilation. Accommodation begins as he explores this idea and thinks about how he learned that the world was flat and begins to compare that with the new information he has been acquiring. This step is closely followed by incorporating the new information in a way that allows him to create growth. He might create balance by recognizing that he believed in the flatness of the world due to the information he had at the time. It is not about stupidity or stubbornness, but simply a lack of information. He is then able to see how he is growing in knowledge and can feel excited about this new round-world discovery. This process is how we all learn and develop.

Erikson

Erik Erikson, another psychologist known for his work in developmental theory, suggests that we are faced with tasks of development, akin to forks in the road on the path to maturity. Our environments, experiences, and perceptions affect us as we approach various developmental tasks. Erikson lists eight developmental tasks, including such areas as the development of trust versus mistrust, autonomy versus shame and doubt, intimacy versus isolation, and integrity versus despair. This theoretical approach is important in a discussion of DID because it offers a wonderful road map for ascertaining where trauma is likely to have occurred. In infancy, for example, a child learns whether the world is trustworthy based on the experiences of his little environment. At this time of life, abandonment or separation anxiety issues are likely to develop if caretakers are abusive or simply unavailable for some reason. If one of a person's issues is a fear of abandonment, it is probably related to this stage of development, in which nurturing from a caretaker was so vital. Attachment theory, described below, also speaks to this developmental issue. As a baby, a child is helpless and depends on the adults in her life for her very survival, but sometimes those adults are neglectful or have limits of their own that prevented healthy interaction. A mother who is dissociative might pick up her crying infant, but if she is in a dissociated state herself, it is highly unlikely that she will be able to provide comforting that is connected. The baby picks up on this disconnection and learns not to expect too much from the mother in terms of emotional connectedness. She may even begin to mirror the mother's behavior. As an adult, however, she is likely to continue to search for that connection with a mother figure. At some level, she understands that something is missing in her relationships.

Bowlby and Ainsworth

> Throughout adult life the availability of a responsive attachment figure remains the source of a person's feeling secure.
> (John Bowlby)

Attachment theory, developed by John Bowlby and Mary Ainsworth, is especially important to a discussion of DID. Simply put, attachment theory is concerned with the relationship that occurs between children and their primary caregivers. The importance of attachment is that it creates an environment in which a child can begin to explore safely, knowing that the caregiver will remain constant. This relationship is referred to as a "secure base." The example of the mother picking up her crying infant while in a dissociated state herself illustrates how healthy attachment can be thwarted.

Attachment develops in infancy as caregivers interact with a child by providing consistent nurturing responses to the child's behavior. Although attachment is biologically based, it does not develop in a healthy and secure manner without that nurturing environment. As Robert Karen has written, "Researchers now know that 'secure attachment' between infant and mother (or other primary caregiver) is critical to a child's psychological development."[5] Secure attachment provides a child with confidence, a sense of security, and the knowledge that his needs will be met on a consistent basis, all important ingredients in the formation of a solid Self.

In DID, the development of attachment is typically hindered due to abuse, neglect, or inconsistent responses from primary caregivers. As a result, these children learn not to expect consistent nurturing from others. An important component of DID therapy is to address the developmental deficits and attachment issues that were created in childhood. The basis for that work is the relationship the DID client has with the therapist.

DEVELOPMENTAL DEFICITS

Attachment issues are what lie at the core of developmental stages. If something is missed along the way, it is like a huge pothole in the road: what was supposed to be there is missing. When you hit the pothole, you immediately know that something is wrong and it wreaks havoc on your car, but what do you do? You keep on going. So, too, the child who missed that nurturing connection with a caretaker just kept on going. He adapted to the road that was set before him, yet he cannot help but wonder what is missing in relationships with self and others now.

The first five to seven years of life are often referred to as being the most important in terms of development. During the first two years of life, a child moves from complete reliance on a caretaker to learning to operate as a separate human being. Psychologists refer to the process as *individuation*. Parents refer to it as "the terrible twos." The goal is for the parent to allow the child to begin to individuate in a safe way. If a power struggle occurs between parent and child, it is quite likely the child will become overly concerned with perfection or will act in oppositional or passive-aggressive ways. When a child feels that he has to choose between himself and a parent, it creates a no-win situation. Later in life, relationships for that individual may be fraught with power struggles or a splitting defense where people are perceived as either all good or all bad. In DID, these same dynamics are at work. First, there is a fear of abandonment. Second, there is a feeling of having to choose between self and others so as to be a good person. The fear of individuation becomes terrifying.[6]

Ages three to six are the time of life when children begin to learn about social roles and what it means to be male or female within society. It is a period when peer relationships are very important and learning how to get along with others and create a sense of belonging is crucial. This time presents a wonderful teaching opportunity for parents. The trick is to teach without becoming too authoritarian or anxious. In other words, parents need to allow the child to learn through experience so that she will connect with her inner strengths. Many adults with DID did not get the opportunity to develop healthy relationships in childhood because of the chaotic environments in which they were living. When energy is being focused on survival, it is hard to think about interacting with others, and when previous stages have taught a child that the world is unsafe and that people cannot be trusted, it is easy to understand why that same child would enter into relationships with hesitancy. Many adults with DID talk about feeling different from other people, even alien. They learn to play roles and they do it well, but when it comes to interacting socially with others they talk about a deep sense of loneliness that pervades whatever they do. It is the belief that "I do not belong." Worse yet, for some it is the belief that "I do not deserve to belong."

In later chapters, we talk about treatment. The truth is that many people suffer from learning deficits in development; it is simply a matter of degree. Yet like the potholes that are filled and leveled, the deficits can be overcome. The road does not have to be bumpy forever.

These theories provide valuable information about human development and, when woven together, can give insight into the behavior of someone with DID. For the therapist, this insight can be a reminder that behavior is indeed adaptive. Today's behavior is very much related to yesterday and the yesterdays of long ago. It is also related to the human ability to incorporate and adapt to the lessons of experience. That information can help the DID client understand why she gets "stuck" in behaviors that seem so unrelated to chronological age. Concerned persons in the life of an individual with DID can use these theories to remind themselves of their own developmental process and gain more empathy for the ways in which the dissociator's development was thwarted due to neglect or trauma inflicted by others. It reminds us of the extremely important adage, "We're in this together." As human beings, we develop in similar ways. We have many choices to make as we grow, but as children we are not able to choose our environments. The good news is that development that is interrupted can continue to move forward. What is needed is an occasional jump start.

EXAMPLES OF ADAPTIVE FUNCTIONING

- A child is being physically abused. When his father grabs him and starts to beat him, the child backs into the wall and, in his mind, disappears into the wall, which helps him minimize the pain of the abuse.
- A little girl is being sexually abused. Whenever the abuse happens, she sees herself float to the ceiling of her bedroom and another little girl experiences the abuse instead.
- A ten-year-old girl has many fragmented parts due to the trauma she has suffered in her childhood. She has learned that she can "disappear" whenever she feels frightened. What she does not realize is that various inside parts come out to live whenever she disappears, helping her look normal when circumstances feel too overwhelming to deal with.
- An adult woman with DID works in the surgical area of a large hospital. Sometimes, in the middle of the night, she awakens to what she thinks are the footsteps of her father coming down the hall to her bedroom. She dissociates and a younger part comes out, terrified that she is about to be abused. An inside "helper" quickly moves into the

forefront and takes control. She reminds the child that they are no longer in any danger and helps her find a safe place inside where she can go to sleep. The next morning the adult is up and ready for work. Sometimes she remembers being awake at night and other times her only clue is that she feels as though she has had a fitful sleep. Nonetheless, the memory of the previous night stays outside her consciousness until she has finished her busy day with patients.

- Nancy hates sex. Even more likely, she is afraid of it. Sex to her is about power and abuse, not love. Yet she is married to a wonderful, loving man. What can she do to reconcile her feelings about sex and love? The typical cycle starts with a sexual encounter between Nancy and her husband. She is usually fine until something happens to trigger her into a memory of past abuse. It might be the way he breathes on her neck or how he touches her, however tenderly. That creates panic internally for Nancy, so a stronger, more aggressive part comes out who feels better able to handle the situation. Her husband, though, is generally able to detect the switch and it creates distance between them. She adapts to protect herself from painful memories even though it creates problems in her marriage.

- Cindy wants to kill herself every time she has memories of her childhood abuse. Sometimes the memories appear as pictures in her mind, and at other times she feels intense sadness and fear, but something keeps her from hurting herself. She cannot fully explain what happens. All Cindy knows is that she goes into a kind of trance and does not have the energy to hurt herself. Typically, she falls asleep and then wakes up a few hours later feeling capable of dealing with life again. What she does not know is that she has an inside part whose job is to keep her alive.

ADAPTIVE VERSUS MALADAPTIVE FUNCTIONS OF DID

Many functions are served by dissociation, and experts in the trauma field generally agree that DID is in part an adaptive response to trauma. In the case of DID specifically, adaptive dissociation is often used for the purposes listed below. As you read, consider the ways in which these behaviors may function or evolve to include both adaptive and maladaptive features.

Self-Soothing and Numbing

Self-soothing and numbing are ways of creating safety from perceived threats. Numbing occurs when dissociators go into a mild trance state so that they will be less responsive, both physically and emotionally, to what is going on around them. Some dissociators have parts that are especially skilled at creating these states whenever another part becomes self-destructive, which prevents the self-destructive state from acting out in a dangerous way. Numbing can serve as a way of self-soothing, but it is certainly not the only way. With DID, fairly benign situations can be experienced as life threatening due to the flashbacks that can occur. In childhood, the individual with DID experienced high levels of trauma. To survive, she had to invent ways of comforting herself that would not attract a lot of attention from abusers. Self-soothing may have taken place through the behaviors of thumb sucking, rocking, sleeping, or even having internal conversations among parts. Numbing is a more extreme example that can be especially helpful during abuse because it can assist the child to retreat internally and not reveal her fear. Now, when the child has grown up, self-soothing might take on similar forms or more "adult" forms, such as overeating or alcohol and drug abuse. Numbing can certainly occur through those behaviors, but dissociators are also adept at going into trancelike states that allow them to turn the world off, at least momentarily.

Creating Connections with Others

Adults with DID learned at an early age that they were not allowed to have voices of their own. They may have been afraid to form relationships with others due to mistrust, yet they still look for satisfying relationships, as we all do. Until appropriate social skills are learned, creating a crisis or relying on a more charming or social alter may be the way that the connection is created. To rely on a victim stance or an always pleasing personality, however, creates difficulty for other parts and can become manipulative. Such action leaves relationships feeling very one-sided, which actually increases the fear of abandonment. As children, individuals with DID learned to form relationships with others by being very pleasing or by becoming high achievers. Many learned to anticipate the needs of others and developed a caretaking style. As adults, they may continue to play whatever role was most successful in childhood. Adults with DID are very skilled at assessing their surroundings and becoming whatever they believe is expected of them, which creates the illusion of being close to others.

Keeping Abuse Secrets Intact

Perpetrators take advantage of a child's vulnerability and use it to their own advantage. The typical behavior of an abuser is to lie to the child to convince him that the abuse is deserved or that terrible things will happen if anyone is told. The lies may include threats to kill pets or family members. The abuser might also distort the delightful stages children go through when they exhibit magical thinking and a belief in superheroes and fantasy figures such as Santa Claus or the Easter Bunny. It is easy to tease a child and convince him of things that are not true. The abuser uses this ability to ensure that his behavior will never be discovered. Individuals with DID continue to believe the threats. Remember that younger parts may act as though they are stuck in time. Thus, a child part may hold on to the belief that she is in danger if she talks about the abuse. This behavior is extremely adaptive for a child because it can help her to feel safer emotionally by keeping knowledge of the abuse contained in one area of the mind. It becomes dysfunctional in adulthood if the threat no longer exists, however. If a child alter keeps information hidden, the adult will continue to operate in dissociated states of which she may not even be aware. Not only is such behavior retraumatizing, but it could actually be dangerous if a child part emerges when an adult needs to be in charge. Fortunately, when a person begins to trust the therapist, she will become more able to share information about past abuse. Initially, however, some parts may react in anger or fear to keep other parts quiet and to ensure the safety of the system as a whole. In cases in which an abuser has convinced the child to hurt herself if the secret is exposed, it becomes very important for other parts to move in so that a suicidal or homicidal part will not hurt the body. These issues are addressed as a part of therapy.

Managing Emotions

There are two primary reasons individuals with DID feel overwhelmed by their feelings. One is that they experienced overwhelming feelings as the result of trauma, and their developing brains were not able to cope with the stimuli. As adults, they may still continue to suffer from PTSD symptoms. Another common experience is that parts were created to deal with various emotions. In fact, it is even common for these parts to be named for specific emotions. Now, as adults, they may continue to relegate the expression of those emotions to particular parts because it feels too overwhelming to deal with them in any other way. If today's sadness is carried by a child ego state answering to the name of "Sad" or "The Hurt One," problems are bound to follow. First, the child alter will be trying to manage an adult emotion or situation that she will not be equipped to handle. Second, the child alter, who is stuck in time or operating in concrete thought, will be approaching both the problem and the solution through a child's eyes. Third, the strong emotion might be triggering for the child ego state, causing her to react as though she is in extreme danger rather than experiencing a feeling called sadness. This example shows why learning to manage emotions effectively is an essential therapy goal for someone with DID.

Performing Daily Roles and Functions

Alters may have also been developed to deal with various functions in life. Maybe one part goes to work, another part does the parenting, and another fulfills social obligations. Because parts are compartmentalized, it makes sense that they would want to function in the world in a compartmentalized fashion as well. For someone with DID, compartmentalizing can be an excellent way of performing roles efficiently and with a minimal amount of stress. In fact, dissociators are sometimes able to accomplish more than those who are integrated because of this ability to compartmentalize. Some people even report being able to do more than one task at a time because different parts are able to focus on different tasks.

Self-Punishment and Reenactment of Abuse

People with DID usually have one or more parts who believe that they are bad and deserve to be punished. Sometimes abusers tell them these things. Sometimes it is a self-adopted belief that bad things only happen to bad people. Consequently, when a mistake is made or life becomes more stressful than usual, the individual will direct blame toward herself. Self-punishment becomes a way of relieving the emotional distress. For others, it is a kind of penance for absolving shame. For yet others, it is an unconscious way of doing what was done to them, a learned response, a kind of self-sabotage that demonstrates to the world that they feel unworthy of life.

Creating Safety

The most typical way of creating internal safety is to dissociate and allow the most capable alter for the situation to emerge. That can happen in myriad ways, be it an angry alter who keeps everyone safe when feeling threatened by someone or an alter who numbs the system to keep another part from committing suicide. As therapy progresses, the system will begin to learn to work together, in a more conscious way, to create safety and learn to tolerate a wide range of emotion.

Reinforcement of Misbeliefs about Self and Others

Individuals with DID share many common beliefs about themselves and the world. Some of the beliefs, such as, "I am a bad person and deserved to be abused," are untrue. Others, however, may be based

QUESTIONS FOR REFLECTION

For Those Who Experience Dissociation

1. How has DID been adaptive in your life? Make a list of specific ways that DID has helped you to survive. In what ways has DID become maladaptive in your life? List specific problems you deal with as a result of being a person with DID.
2. What role does dissociation play in your life at this particular point in time? What keeps you from functioning effectively?
3. Who knows that you have DID? How can you get support from these people? Make a list of their names and phone numbers and keep a copy with you in case of an emergency.
4. When thinking about the adaptive function of DID, some people find it helpful to list internal parts and describe their function or role. You might want to do that here.

Example	Name of Internal Part	Function
	Sally, age five	Holds the frightening memories of a specific incident of abuse. Carries the feeling of fear.
	Marcy, age twelve	The pleaser. Able to keep others calm, which in turn helps little ones feel safer on the inside.

partially in truth. A person may hold the belief that "men cannot be trusted" because she was abused by a male caretaker. Although some men are not trustworthy, the generalized belief that no man can be trusted is simply not true, but the part who holds such a belief will act as though it is true. So, it is conceivable that one part could be pursuing a relationship with a man, while another (based on *her*

QUESTIONS FOR REFLECTION, *continued*

For Therapists

1. Assess your own beliefs about DID. Do you consider it to be a mental illness, an attachment/developmental disorder, or an example of adaptive functioning? Why?

2. What are your reasons for wanting to treat DID? How do you keep the client's best interest in mind? Give specific examples.

3. List as many ways as you can think of that DID has been helpful to your client's survival.

4. What do you see your client doing to function effectively? How can you encourage your client to continue to develop those skills?

5. What skills or behaviors does your client need that he or she is currently lacking?

For Concerned Persons

1. Are you able to appreciate what the DID person in your life has done to survive? What can you say and do to show your support?

2. List as many ways as you can think of that DID has helped your loved one to survive.

3. What does your friend or loved one do to function in daily life? If you are not sure, do you want to ask her if she is willing to share more with you? Why or why not?

4. How do you feel about having someone in your life with DID? Be honest about the positives and negatives of such a relationship.

---

beliefs) is doing things to push the man away. We all create beliefs about ourselves in relationship to the rest of the world. Our behaviors will then fall in line with those beliefs, true or not, until we stop long enough to ask ourselves which of the beliefs are truly healthy and based on reality.

SUMMARY

If the behaviors of someone with DID are adaptive, why would treatment be needed? The answer is that adaptation can be progressive, so behavior that was useful at one time may need to be modified if it is to continue being helpful. The goals of therapy with DID clients vary, but all are geared toward helping the person function effectively in life and in an integrated, or conscious, fashion. The coping skills previously mentioned are based in part on past experiences and distorted beliefs. Dissociation is a means of survival, but if an individual continues to live as though the past and the present are the same, their quality of life will be greatly diminished. When that happens, what was once adaptive becomes *maladaptive*.

In the next chapter, we discuss treatment options. First, though, reflect on the questions on pages 52 and 53. Create a space in which you can think about what DID means to your own life.

Chapter Three

Diagnosing the Disorder

Nancy had struggled with depression and eating disorders for years. Her treatment had consisted of both individual therapy and inpatient programs, yet nothing seemed to work. As her life became more and more out of control, she called a friend and begged for help. Nancy's description of her life pointed to the possibility of a dissociative disorder. She talked about losing time and occasionally "waking up" in dangerous situations and not knowing how she got there. When people asked questions about her childhood, she felt confused and unable to provide specific answers. As she began to look at her journal entries over the years, there were distinct changes in the handwriting, yet no therapist had caught the dissociative piece. Instead, everyone focused on Nancy's eating disorder, not understanding why there was never any improvement. Was it that she just didn't want to get better?

Nancy's experience with the mental health system is not unusual for someone who is dealing with a dissociative disorder. In fact, most DID patients see several therapists and have an average of seven diagnoses before finally finding someone who understands the dissociative aspect of their behavior.[1] Part of the reason for this problem is that too few therapists are trained in the diagnosis and treatment of DID. Furthermore, many therapists do not believe in the existence of the disorder, despite its inclusion in the *DSM-IV,* the diagnostic manual used by mental health professionals. For someone like Nancy, that may mean years of ineffective treatment.

Confirming the diagnosis of DID is not easy, however. One of the difficulties lies in the nature of dissociation, which compartmentalizes behaviors and experience that would normally be connected. Also, the dissociative personality system is usually set up to avoid detection. As with every diagnostic category, however, clues can point a person in the right direction. Clues can help because the diagnosis and treatment of DID is much like putting together a puzzle of a person's life, albeit with a few missing pieces along the way.

> I was in therapy for two and a half years, treating DID, but had been in therapy for approximately thirteen years prior to that diagnosis. Originally, it was for depression. It was my family doctor who referred me to a specialist in treating DID. Because she did not have the time to take on new patients, she referred me to a therapist who was qualified in dealing with DID. Validating that the abuse did happen has helped me to explain why I have always been so "different."
> (Stephanie, client, Canada)

INDICATORS OF DISSOCIATION

People go to therapy for a variety of reasons. Sometimes it is to deal with situational stress, other times it is to deal with an affective disorder like depression or anxiety, and sometimes it is because life is feeling chaotic and out of control. There are just as many reasons for the person with DID to begin treatment, and there are indicators that dissociation may be an issue. If a client has seen several different therapists yet does not report much progress, screening for dissociation may be indicated. Another clue is a self-report of a chaotic lifestyle that has been pervasive over time, which is likely to be experienced within the therapeutic relationship in the form of missed appointments, abrupt mood changes, and forgetfulness. The most obvious clue is dissociation during the session, even though a therapist may or may not see switching from one state to another early in therapy. Yet these clues are all good indicators of a dissociative problem that may present itself in the initial sessions, leading the therapist to investigate further.

As with any client, the therapist will begin by asking the client why she is there and what she hopes to accomplish with therapy. An accurate social, psychiatric, and physical history will provide the initial clues that dissociation might be an issue. In the initial sessions, therapists generally try to learn about family dynamics and whether any abuse occurred directly or indirectly within the family. Even if other parts carry memories of abuse and are not immediately forthcoming with the information, clients may still talk about relationships or behaviors within the family that appear normal to the client but that the therapist recognizes as examples of abuse, neglect, or disorganized attachment. Therapists, however, rarely confront these issues directly until they have developed a strong therapeutic relationship with the client.

It is perfectly appropriate for therapists to ask clients if they were abused in childhood, and it is also appropriate to name behaviors as abusive, even if the client disagrees with that assessment. It is not appropriate, however, for a therapist to try to convince a client that she has been abused if she believes that she has not, even if the client's denial appears to have more to do with her dissociation than with reality. Nor is it appropriate for a therapist to suggest to a client that she needs to undergo hypnosis or take drugs, such as Amytal, solely for the purpose of uncovering repressed memories. Reputable and experienced therapists in the field of dissociation are aware of these limits, but clients need to be aware of them as well. It is a client's right to expect good therapy.

Part of the family of origin information that the client and therapist will need to explore is the issue of rules and consequences, such as who enforced the discipline, how it was enforced, and how family conflicts were resolved. Issues related to alcoholism or other addictions will often enter the conversation at this point. This information will help to form a picture of the family system and the way it operated. The client's beliefs about conflict and how affection was displayed in the family also need to be explored. Some people do not have an adequate understanding of the concept of nurturing and healthy attachment to a caregiver because it did not occur consistently within their own families. Consequently, the client may not have a strong sense of how to feel safe in the world. All this information provides direction in terms of what might be addressed first in therapy. In the initial interview stage, the therapist may or may not know that the client is dissociative, nor will the therapist necessarily be looking for it. The initial goal will be to take a thorough history to determine the most likely direction to proceed diagnostically.

Other indicators present in this interview that might point toward DID are periods of amnesia for parts of the individual's childhood as well as amnesia that occurs currently, referred to as dissociative amnesia. Clients may make statements such as, "I have a really bad memory" or "I do not remember much before the age of [pick a number]." Dissociative clients often provide the therapist with conflictive information, such as "Oh yeah, I had tons of friends while growing up." Then, in the next breath, they might say something such as "I always felt so lonely when I was a child. I was never included in things." Or, a client will report that one year he was an A student, and the next year he was failing, but he does not have a reasonable explanation why.

DID VERSUS SCHIZOPHRENIA

Another important aspect in diagnosis is what Colin Ross refers to as the multiplicity triad.[2] The elements of this triad include that dissociators generally score positively in symptoms typically considered to be indicators of schizophrenia. These symptoms include such things as believing that their thoughts, feelings, or actions are being controlled by something outside of themselves. They also include beliefs that others can hear their thoughts, that thoughts are being taken out of their minds, or that voices are commenting on their actions. These symptoms all represent a third of the triad. The other aspects of the triad include hearing internal voices and reporting past suicide attempts. The major distinguishing factor between DID and schizophrenia, however, is that dissociators hear voices from within themselves and do not lose touch with reality, as occurs with psychosis. Even though someone may be living with DID, he is probably experiencing the internal voices as a *part* of himself. Many dissociators say that they have lived with internal voices for as long as they can remember and are actually surprised to learn that other people do not. (See Table 3.1.)

Additional information helpful in diagnosis is a thorough physical history. Dissociators often report having lifelong physical symptoms that are unexplainable, most notably stomachaches, headaches that are typically diagnosed as migraines, and urinary tract problems. Other common complaints include aversions to certain foods and a gag reflex that may be indicative of oral sex, choking, or some other type of physical assault in childhood.[3]

EGO STATES AND DIAGNOSIS

When a client enters therapy with a prior diagnosis, it might be difficult for the therapist to think outside of the box that has been presented. One reason a dissociative individual might have several different diagnoses, however, is that as different parts present, they may also be presenting with diagnostic issues that are different from the host. Such differences especially make sense given the nature of

Table 3.1 Review of Symptoms in the Context of Schizophrenia and Dissociative Identity Disorder (DID)

Symptoms Characteristic of Schizophrenia	Overlapping Symptoms Potentially Present in Both Schizophrenia and DID	Symptoms Characteristic of DID
Usually isolated symptoms (none to mild severity ratings on the SCID-D, rev.*). Symptoms occur in the context of bizarre delusions or other psychotic symptoms.	Dissociative symptoms	Recurrent to persistent dissociative symptoms (moderate to severe severity ratings on the SCID-D, rev.*)
Lack of sense of identity and one's role in society.	Identity confusion/disturbance	Recurrent and consistent alterations in one's identity.
Hallucinations other than voices of alter personalities. These hallucinations are perceived as occurring primarily outside the patient's head.	Auditory hallucinations and internal dialogues	Auditory hallucinations reflect dialogues between alter personalities. These voices are perceived as occurring inside the patient's head. Often described as similar to thoughts.
Bizarre delusions, paranoid delusions, and any other delusions that do not involve the other personalities, such as, "The CIA is out to get me."	Schneiderian symptoms and delusions	Only delusions are "delusions of several personalities" or of other bodily changes representative of the different personalities.

	Other psychotic symptoms	Absent in DID.
Thinking characterized by incoherence or marked loosening of associations		
Catatonic behavior.		Absent in DID.
Chronic flat affect.		Absent in DID.
Impaired reality testing.	Reality testing	Intact reality testing; "as if" descriptions of dissociative symptoms are typical.
"If mood episodes have occurred during active-phase symptoms, their total duration has been brief relative to the duration of the active and residual periods" (DSM-IV, pp. 284–86).	Comorbid diagnoses	The full depressive or manic syndrome may coexist with the dissociative syndrome.

*Structured Clinical Interview for DSM-IV Dissociative Disorders, revised

Continued overleaf

Table 3.1 Schneiderian Symptoms Normally Associated with Schizophrenia, *continued*

Symptoms Characteristic of Schizophrenia	Overlapping Symptoms Potentially Present in Both Schizophrenia and DID	Symptoms Characteristic of DID
"One or more areas of functioning, such as work, interpersonal, relations, or self-care are markedly below the level achieved prior to the onset" (*DSM-IV*, p. 285).	Impairment in functioning	Any impairment in functioning is usually temporary, with eventual full return to premorbid level of functioning.
"Continuous signs of the disturbance for at least 6 months" (*DSM-IV*, p. 285).	Course of symptoms and syndrome	Signs of the disturbance may be intermittent. Rapid fluctuations in symptoms, mood, and degree of impairment may occur.

Reprinted with permission from the *Interviewer's Guide to the Structured Clinical Interview for DSM-IV Dissociative Disorders*. Revised by Marlene Steinberg, M.D. copyright 1994 American Psychiatric Press, Inc.

DID. When experiences or emotions become too overwhelming, the mind cleverly encapsulates the material and stores it for safe-keeping. Many people respond this way in the face of trauma, but the additional step that occurs in this process, in the case of DID, is the formation of distinct ego states that carry the experience. Because one of the criteria necessary for the diagnosis of DID is "the presence of two or more distinct personalities (each with its own relatively enduring pattern of perceiving, relating to, and thinking about the environment and self)," it becomes easier to understand how different diagnoses can occur in the same individual. One part might present as depressed, whereas another presents as anxious. This difference can create confusion diagnostically if the therapist is not aware of the dissociative piece.

Suppose that one part has learned to react to threats in the environment by becoming extremely anxious to the point that she worries about most things in her life, has headaches and stomachaches associated with the anxiety, and is experiencing fatigue, difficulty concentrating, and irritability. Consequently, she receives a diagnosis of generalized anxiety disorder. Then, another part presents who has dealt with the stress of life by shutting down. As a child, she learned that this behavior was the way to stay alive. So now, when life feels like it is too much to bear, she becomes isolated and withdrawn, begins to have suicidal thoughts, and complains of a poor appetite, difficulty sleeping, and feelings of hopelessness. Based on her presentation and the length of time she has been experiencing the symptoms, the client may receive a diagnosis of depression. Another part, very likely stuck developmentally in adolescence, may act out to manage her stress. She uses alcohol and bingeing and purging behavior as a way to manage feelings and does so very well. Yet to the unsuspecting therapist who, up to now, has seen only the host personality, this new behavior may seem very alarming and out of character. Now the client has a diagnosis of bulimia and, maybe, substance abuse. Now we have one person and three diagnoses, actually four if you count the host personality and whatever diagnosis she has been carrying throughout therapy.

BORDERLINE PERSONALITY DISORDER VERSUS DID

One of the most prevalent diagnostic issues encountered when assessing dissociation is DID and its relationship with borderline personality disorder (BPD). It is very common for dissociators to be diagnosed as BPD at some point in their therapy careers. Let's briefly look at what constitutes BPD so that we can discuss why BPD and DID are so often intertwined.

BPD is a personality disorder characterized by frantic attempts to avoid abandonment (real or imagined), unstable relationships with a tendency to view people as either all good or all bad, impulsivity that is often related to substance use or sexual behavior, recurrent suicidal attempts or self-mutilation, and inappropriate displays of anger.

Persons with DID may look borderline due to switching behavior among ego states. If the therapist is not aware of what is happening, the client's behavior will seem very confusing. In a childlike state, a client may fear being abandoned by the therapist and may make frantic phone calls to make sure that the therapist is available, not angry with her, and so on. In one state, the client may like the therapist and feel very attached, in another state she might feel angry with the therapist and disconnected, and in yet another state she might feel anxious about the security of the relationship, all at the same time. Imagine the confusion a therapist might feel if these states all occur in a single session. Then suppose that the therapist tries to confront the issue to better understand what is happening, but instead of reaching some mutual understanding about the situation, the client ends up feeling attacked. The client then gets drunk on the way home because she feels as though the therapist has rejected her.

Such situations are not uncommon when treating clients who are DID or BPD. Even if the diagnosis is clearly DID, it is reasonable to pay attention to borderline behaviors that alert the therapist to treatment issues or to a better understanding of the client's internal personality structure. It is inappropriate for therapists to use BPD as a wastebasket diagnosis, which some do, for clients who present with difficult behaviors or symptoms. It may be appropriate, however, to diagnose both DID and BPD in the same individual if the criteria are clearly met for both.[4]

There are disagreements in the therapeutic community about the classification of BPD as a personality disorder, and some therapists believe BPD could be treated more effectively if it were categorized as a dissociative disorder, along with DID.[5] The reasons are varied. First, BPD is thought by many to develop in response to abuse or neglect in childhood. Second, there is a dissociative component to BPD. The dissociative episodes tend to be more transient in nature than with DID, but there is dissociation nonetheless. There are distinct mood changes with borderline individuals that may be experienced as very alien or disconnected to the client. The loss of memory associated with DID, however, does not occur in BPD, and the mood changes do not constitute a change in personality to the extent that a part of the psyche takes control of the body outside the individual's consciousness.

BPD's classification as a personality disorder has, unfortunately, led some therapists, and most insurance companies, to take the position that these individuals never change. Often, however, the dissociative aspect of the disorder has never been addressed, although it is crucial to successful treatment. Fortunately, since the development of Marsha Linehan's dialectical behavioral therapy (DBT), persons with BPD are beginning to be treated in a more effective and respectful manner. (We look more closely at DBT when we discuss adjunct therapies in chapter 6). Considering BPD as another possible dissociative diagnosis could help therapists differentiate between that and DID better and enable clients to receive more effective treatment.

EARLY DIAGNOSTIC BENCHMARKS

As previously stated, DID should be considered in anyone who has had several different diagnoses over time. Other issues that may present themselves in the search for the most appropriate diagnosis include physical symptoms. For example, when operating in one ego state, a client may have a physical disorder or illness that other states do not experience. Some medical tests have even been reported to produce varied results for different personalities.[6] Physical symptoms do not always play a primary role in diagnosis, but therapists need to be aware of them because research shows that *somatoform dissociation* is one way both animals and humans react to trauma.[7] Although it is important to have a doctor rule out any suspected illnesses, an understanding of how the client's internal system operates will help the therapist begin to piece together the various stories that the alters share. If the therapist is not aware of the issues associated with dissociative disorders, she may believe she is dealing only with a somatoform disorder in which psychological factors play a major role in the physical symptoms displayed by the patient. DID clients often complain of chronic undiagnosable pain and symptoms such as headaches, visual disturbances, stomachaches, irritable bowel syndrome, urinary tract disorders, and nausea.[8] This statement is not to suggest that psychological factors are unrelated to the physical symptoms experienced by many multiples, but the explanation may be different for those with DID as opposed to some other disorders. In DID, physical symptoms often represent flashbacks, dissociation, or switching among states. If close attention is paid to bodily reactions, they too will provide valuable information about the internal system and how it operates. Severe headaches are especially indicative of switching or internal conflicts among parts.

Additional issues that could point to a diagnosis of DID include reports of inner voices (which differ from the voices of schizophrenia); frequent nightmares beginning in childhood; panic attacks; differences in handwriting; distinct differences in a client's voice, appearance, or style of presentation from session to session; and reports of self-injury, including more covert behaviors such as eating disorders and chemical dependency. Self-injurious behaviors such as eating disorders and chemical abuse serve a variety of functions, most importantly as coping mechanisms. Many dissociative clients develop addictions because the chemicals help to control the intensity of flashbacks and to keep emotions at a more tolerable level. Addictions can also serve as a way for clients to express their anger about what has happened to them.

Eating disorders do the same and, in the case of anorexia, may help the client to feel a greater sense of control. Studies about the relationship between eating disorders and sexual abuse have shown that clients with bulimia are more likely to have experienced childhood sexual abuse than those with anorexia.[9] Bulimics are also more likely to develop problems with chemical addiction. There may be a biological explanation for this phenomenon, although it cannot be stated conclusively at this point. In terms of diagnosis, however, it can be helpful to be aware of what the current research suggests. The binge/purge cycle experienced by bulimics works in much the same way as alcohol in keeping feelings outside of conscious awareness. Some clients describe a surreal sense of calm and detachment, similar to dissociation, that occurs after a binge/purge cycle. Other clients talk about feeling triggered by intense anger that they do not feel they can express in any other way.

Another issue with both chemical dependency and eating disorders is that they serve as ways of harming the self or of expressing one's internal self-loathing to the outside world. Viewed in this way, both behaviors might be considered a form of passive suicide, but they can both be seen as protective coping mechanisms as well. If a particular part carries the diagnosis of chemical dependency or bulimia, that part might be using the behavior as a way to protect the system (usually the host) from pain she does not believe the host can handle. If she is able to numb the pain by using food or alcohol, she has done her job. Keeping the host numb can also serve as a way of keeping system secrets intact by pushing memories farther into the subconscious and focusing time and attention on the addictive behavior.

BASK MODEL

An understanding of Bennett Braun's model can also be helpful during the initial diagnostic phase.[10] Part of the confusion for therapists in the initial stage of therapy is client reporting of information that just does not seem to "add up." Braun's BASK model illustrates how traumatic memory and later recall can occur, or fail to occur, in the areas of behavior, affect, sensation, or knowledge. In dissociative disorders, all four areas tend to be affected to varying degrees. It is not unusual for a client to be missing information in one or more of these areas when reporting a memory, which is what leads to confusion about whether the experience is valid. DID clients often doubt their own memories and may look to the therapist to determine what is and is not true.

> Denial of trauma is abusive to the victim. It is useful to deal with the meaning of possible memories and not try to determine their veracity.
>
> (Judy, therapist, New York)

Client Presentation

A typical client scenario may include spontaneous flashbacks, partial memories, child parts who have been threatened into keeping silent, and an adult who may be fearful of being disbelieved, discredited, or labeled. It is inappropriate for therapists to attempt to verify whether memories are true, because they have no way of doing so. Instead, a competent therapist will take the information, regardless of the channel in which it is presented, and consider it to be another piece of the puzzle. A trauma specialist, Dr. Bessel van der Kolk, has stated that "the body keeps the score."[11] If a client reports bodily sensations or spontaneous flashbacks with corresponding emotion, it is important to validate whatever is being presented. In terms of diagnosis, the client is speaking through his or her symptoms. If a girl experienced abuse in the woods on an autumn day at the age of nine and goes walking in the woods on an autumn day thirty years later, she may experience physical reactions similar to what was experienced during the original abuse. In the case of DID, however, until enough system work has been done in therapy, the adult will probably be at a loss to explain her experience. In terms of the BASK model, she may report affect and sensation related to the past experience, but be unable to put it into the context of a complete narrative.

> I felt anxious as I was walking through the woods and began to smell smoke and immediately thought I was going to vomit. Yet it was a beautiful day and I was with friends. I had the faintest recollection of something bad happening to me in those woods, but I do not know how that could even be possible. I even mentioned the smoke to the others, but they couldn't smell it. Where is this coming from?
> (Susan, client, Minnesota)

With any clinical interview, the therapist's observational skills will affect the accuracy of the final diagnosis. With DID, facial changes and fluctuations in voice and speech patterns offer important data. These changes tend to be more dramatic, or unsettling, than with the typical therapy client. The most obvious changes occur when an adult "switches" and begins to take on the mannerisms and vocal characteristics of a child. At other times, a dissociator might react with extreme fear to something that is benign, like the sound of someone's voice in the hall outside the therapist's office. Or, a client might respond quite angrily to an innocent question posed by the therapist. The response may seem so out of character for the client or so removed from the context of the conversation that the therapist may be confused, if not even thrown a bit off balance, by the client's reaction. In some cases, the client's startle response is so active that she might jump with a look of terror because the therapist "looked at her wrong." All these responses are related to internal switching that is occurring. Amnesia during the session, however slight, is also a high indicator of dissociation and is almost always associated with switching.

I was talking to Jason about the stress he was feeling with his family. He mentioned the lack of communication, the way they skirted around issues that might create even the least bit of conflict. I asked where he had gotten the message that conflict is bad. In an instant, he was commenting on the wood in my desk. At first I found myself feeling a bit agitated. Was this a ploy to get me off the subject? I steered the conversation back to communication issues within the family as soon as I could. As we finished our discussion, I asked Jason why he had been so interested in my desk earlier. He looked at me quizzically and said he didn't know what I was talking about.

I'd guess that we had talked for five or ten minutes about that crazy desk and he wasn't aware of any of the conversation.
(Greg, therapist, Minnesota)

A therapist might suspect amnesia or avoidance if a client looks confused and asks for a question to be repeated or if a therapist asks a client to respond and the client is unable to do so. In these cases, clients often say, "I am sorry, I guess I am really tired" or they might look sleepy or confused and ask for the question to be repeated. At other times, a client might switch in the middle of a conversation and start talking about something else, then switch back and pick up the original conversation where it had been left off. Any therapist inquiries about the switch may be met with confusion or anger if the client is not aware of the switch taking place. During the diagnostic stage of treatment, these changes tend to be subtler, which is why observation is so important. As treatment progresses and switching and the accompanying amnesia increases, the management of these behaviors will become a focus of treatment.

Frank Putnam states that the typical DID diagnosis is made six months after the initial interview.[12] Although this situation may be partially due to therapist unfamiliarity with the disorder, client presentation is also a key factor. One of the functions of DID is to keep the alters hidden and to preserve the internal system, which may also occur in therapy until a degree of trust has been built with the therapist.

According to Colin Ross, the typical DID client is a female, age twenty to forty, with a history of abuse. She will report having blank spells, voices in her head, or other symptoms more commonly associated with schizophrenia (discussed earlier in this chapter); the *DSM* criteria is met or nearly met for BPD; she will have had previous unsuccessful treatment; she will report self-destructive behaviors and chronic headaches, but without the presence of a thought disorder.[13]

Diagnostic Tools

Regardless of the diagnosis, if dissociation is present, it is important to explore what role it is playing in the client's life. Dissociation is a defense. It is important for the therapist to name the dissociation and to talk about defenses in a way that helps to normalize the behavior. The therapist will then begin to work with the client to explore reasons why she might be using this particular defense. If the therapist broaches the subject of dissociation with the client as soon as she becomes aware of it, that will help in terms of diagnosis. Using the dissociative experiences scale (DES) or the somatoform dissociation questionnaire (SDQ-20) at this point may help determine the degree and function of the dissociation as well.

DISSOCIATIVE
EXPERIENCE SCALE (DES)

The DES, developed by Frank Putnam and Eve Carlson, is a self-report measure that helps therapists better understand the frequency of the client's dissociative experiences. Especially helpful about the scale is reliability information to assess the type of dissociation that is occurring. It is important to keep in mind that dissociation does not automatically mean a diagnosis of DID. Knowing when the client is most likely to dissociate, the form that the dissociation takes, and the severity of the dissociation will aid in making a correct diagnosis. As therapists begin to understand the ways in which clients dissociate, they will have solid information that can be explored fully. Talking openly about the behavior gives the client permission to consciously acknowledge it.

SOMATOFORM DISSOCIATION
QUESTIONNAIRE (SDQ-20)

The SDQ-20, developed by Ellert Nijenhuis, measures somatoform dissociation, a frequently overlooked element of dissociation. Somatoform dissociation is associated with physical responses that can occur when people are severely traumatized and the emotions are not expressed on a conscious level. This defensive response is related to behaviors that occur with animals when they are frightened, with freezing being the dominant state. Dissociation allows humans to freeze and develop physical analgesia when threatened, as well. The use of the SDQ-20 can help therapists assess for dissociation and make sense of the unexplainable physical complaints that many dissociative clients present.[14]

It is safe to assume that most client dissociation has developed as a response to some type of trauma in the individual's life. Unless the trauma was very recent, as with a mugging or a car accident, however, it is doubtful that the behavior is truly adaptive in the present. Instead, it has probably become a habitual way of defending, both biologically and psychologically. Dissociators tend to respond in this way before stopping to see if the perceived threat is real. Several broad areas related to this behavior need to be discussed with the client in an exploratory, information-seeking manner. Is the dissociation a learned response that has been present for most of the client's life? Is there any kind of unconscious secondary gain associated with the behavior, such as not having to take responsibility for some aspect of life? Is there an underlying fear that prevents the client from giving up the behavior, such as not feeling strong enough to deal with emotions? Is it simply a matter of not knowing any other way to deal with emotion?

It is important for the therapist to prepare the client somewhat before asking these questions so that the client does not feel unduly threatened. If not, the client may be pushed farther into the use of the defense. The therapist must continue to normalize the behavior and make very clear to the client the importance of working together to gather the information to help both the therapist and the client better understand the issues being presented. The questioning is not about judging, shaming, or attempting to force change. Although the diagnostic interview will probably cover more than one session, it is an important part of the treatment process. It is vital in terms of developing trust and rapport in the therapeutic relationship to stay within the bounds of the interview rather than moving too quickly to subsequent stages of treatment. Whenever a client is dissociative, there are issues of trust and powerlessness present, and it is important for the therapist to respect that as therapy begins to move forward.

GUIDELINES FOR DIAGNOSIS AND TREATMENT

The International Society for the Study of Dissociation (ISSD) has developed general guidelines for the diagnosis and treatment of DID. It states that the foundation for diagnosis is a mental status exam that focuses on questions related to dissociative symptoms. The ISSD also recommends the use of dissociative screening instruments, such as the DES (discussed earlier in this chapter), the dissociative disorders interview schedule (DDIS), and the structured clinical interview for *DSM-IV* dissociative disorders, revised (SCID-D-R). The complete guidelines are available from the ISSD, and the address is provided in appendix B.

The DDIS, developed by Ross, is a highly structured interview that covers issues related to the diagnosis of DID as well as other psychological disorders. It is helpful in terms of differential diagnosis and provides therapists with the average scores in each subsection based on a sampling of DID clients who have completed the inventory.

The SCID-D-R, developed by Marlene Steinberg, is another highly structured interview instrument used for diagnosing dissociation.[15] An important aspect of Steinberg's work is her identification of five core dissociative symptoms that must be present to diagnose a client with DID or DDNOS. These symptoms are dissociative amnesia, depersonalization, derealization, identity confusion, and identity alteration. DID is experienced by the dissociator as identity confusion, whereas the nondissociator typically experiences life in a more integrated manner. This experience is compounded by the dissociator often feeling disconnected from the world around him, as if living in a dream at times. The SCID-D-R helps the clinician identify the specific aspects of this experience.

There is disagreement among mental health professionals about the use of other diagnostic tools, such as the Minnesota Multiphasic Personality Inventory (MMPI) for diagnosing DID. Typically, with DID clients the MMPI yields results such as an elevated F (validity scale) and an elevated Sc (schizophrenia scale). Although the MMPI is routinely used for diagnosis, it is quite common for DID clients to appear as polysymptomatic and highly disturbed in the test results.[16] These results are often then interpreted by clinicians as indicative of schizophrenia or an axis II personality disorder, such as BPD. Some clinicians are wary of using the MMPI for the diagnosis of DID for those reasons. If the inventory is used, more accurate information can be gleaned by administering the recently developed MMPI-2.

With the development of structured interviews such as the DDIS and SCID-D-R, dissociative screening devices such as the DES and SDQ-20, and a clearer understanding of the signs and symptoms associated with DID, most therapists are able to diagnosis the disorder accurately as the therapeutic relationship progresses.

Nonetheless, the therapist's basic components related to the diagnostic process include, but are not limited to, the following:

A Thorough History
- An initial interview ranging from one to three sessions.
- Special emphasis given to family of origin issues as well as physical and psychiatric history, with the therapist noting gaps in memory or inconsistencies in client reporting.

Direct Observation
- Taking note of amnesia and avoidance that is occurring within the session.
- Noticing changes in facial features or voice quality that seem out of context to the situation or what is being reported.
- Noting extreme sleepiness or confusion that interferes with the client's ability to track with the therapist during the session.

Screening for Dissociation
- If dissociation is suspected, using a screening tool such as the DES, DDIS, SDQ-20, or SCID-D-R to gather more information.
- Noting symptoms related to amnesia, depersonalization, derealization, identity confusion, and identity alteration before making a diagnosis of DID or DDNOS.

Differential Diagnosis to Rule Out Specific Disorders
- Considering previous diagnoses first; that is, taking into account the number of diagnoses, how many times the client has been treated, and whether past treatments have been successful. Previous diagnoses will be considered, but not used, unless DSM criterion is currently met.

- Comparing DSM criterion for each disorder that has dissociation as a part of its makeup and diagnosing DID only after observing switching among ego states.
- If substance abuse or eating disorders are present and dissociation is suspected, using dissociative screening tools in addition to diagnostic measures that would normally be used for CD or ED assessment to help obtain a more accurate picture regarding the function of the dissociation.

Confirming the Diagnosis
- If dissociation is confirmed, again comparing the DSM criterion for possible diagnoses and diagnosing DID only after observing switching among ego states. Until that time, DDNOS or PTSD may be the more accurate diagnosis.

SUMMARY

The assessment and diagnosis of DID is a process that is sometimes completed within the first few sessions or, more often, that extends into the first stage of treatment. Dissociation can be difficult to diagnose because dissociative clients often enter therapy in a state of crisis. Certainly, stabilization and creating psychological and physical safety for a client is more important than diagnosis, which is why the initial treatment and assessment phases often overlap. The following chapters discuss the stages of therapy with a DID client, specific treatment techniques, and when to implement them. The information presented in these chapters is introductory and general in nature. The diagnosis and treatment of DID should be done by a therapist with an appropriate level of training or by someone in consultation with a clinician who is more experienced.

Chapter Four

Treatment Philosophies and Approaches

Tina's mind had become flooded with memories of childhood abuse. Surprisingly, these memories were beginning to have feelings attached to them, which was new for her. The internal voices were talking constantly, and Tina began to feel a sense of panic that was beyond anything she had known before. In her own mind, the solution was easy enough. Take a handful of Valium, drink enough vodka to block out the din of the voices, pass out, and start over again the following day. The end result of Tina's "self-help" plan, though, was a twenty-eight-day stay in a residential chemical dependency program. She left the program with an aftercare plan that included individual therapy for sexual abuse. Although she agreed with the plan, there were questions churning away inside. "How do I even begin to look for a therapist?" "Where on earth will I get the money?"

INSURANCE VERSUS FEE FOR SERVICE

Tina's questions are actually very realistic. Health care is based primarily on the medical model, even in the area of mental health, with insurance companies requiring a diagnosis based on pathology. This requirement in turn creates a paper trail of diagnoses for the client that can create difficulties when applying for insurance and possibly even jobs in the future. If clients do not use their insurance plans, however, how can they expect to afford long-term treatment? This written record, coupled with too few therapists being trained in the treatment of DID, creates a dilemma for clients before they even walk through a therapist's door.

One of the first decisions that people have to make when starting therapy is whether to use insurance to pay for services. In the current climate of managed care treatment, certain issues have to be considered. Financially, it is certainly more feasible to use insurance benefits than to pay out of pocket, but clients need to be aware that most companies do not offer coverage for long-term care. Thus, a person may start therapy and within the first ten to twenty sessions be told that continued therapy is not medically necessary. This scenario is not always the case, but it can be, and it is important to be aware of the possibility. When issues such as this one arise, the therapist will usually fill out a prior authorization report, which is a request to the insurance company for more hours. In this report, the therapist will review the client's symptoms and how they are interfering with her ability to function. The therapist will also give a diagnosis and discuss the goals of therapy. The client, however, is the one who will need to decide whether she wants the insurance company to have this type of information. Once the information leaves the therapist's office, the ability to control confidentiality is lost. The client will not know who at the insurance company will have access to the information or when doctors, lawyers, or new employers might request information. Granted, release forms have to be signed for medical records to be copied, but can you imagine telling a new employer that you refuse to sign the release? One way around this dilemma is by not allowing the prior authorization initially. It is possible for clients to use insurance until the initial coverage runs out and then pay for services on their own.

Another option is to pay cash from the onset of therapy, which is generally referred to as fee for service. Therapists charge different rates. Sometimes the fee has to do with the typical rate for the area where they practice. Sometimes the fee is established according to degree, licensure, and years of experience. Some therapists even charge according to their own belief systems. For instance, some Christian therapists choose to charge lower fees because they consider their work a ministry. Other therapists are invested in providing affordable fees because the clientele with whom they work—such as single mothers, people living in the inner city, even people with dissociative disorders—may have a difficult time paying for services. In the case of people with DID, finances can become an issue because the client may have seen several therapists before receiving the proper diagnosis. Then, once the diagnosis is made, a client can expect several years of therapy. If money is an issue, one option is to look for someone who charges lower rates or who has a sliding fee scale; that way, a person can pay cash for therapy and not have to worry about prior authorizations and confidentiality issues.

It is important, however, to not be too quick to make assumptions about a therapist based on the charge. First, clients need to seek out therapists who meet their personal criteria for treating the disorder. Then they can begin to compare fees. There are two extremes of thought regarding fees. In accordance with the popular saying "you get what you pay for," do not expect a good therapist to drop fees dramatically. Also, recognize that therapy is a life investment. A person needs to be willing to pay for good treatment. On the other end of the spectrum is the therapist who charges lower-than-normal fees. For some therapists, this policy is truly a humanitarian gesture based on a belief system, but for others it may have more to do with a lack of belief in their own abilities. It is important for clients to take responsibility for their own therapy. Choosing a therapist needs to be based on many things, not just who can be hired at the cheapest rate.

First, narrow the choices, and if one therapist's charges are much higher or lower than the average rate, inquire further. Clients should know why a therapist's rates are different from most others in the area. That information provides valuable insight about the person and who he or she is at a deeper level. Good therapy is based on a partnership between client and therapist. Both need to get to know and respect each other so that they will be able to work together to set lasting, beneficial goals. The relationship begins with the first phone call.

CHOOSING A THERAPIST

Of course, choosing a therapist is based on more than financial concerns. Once someone has decided to enter therapy, how does that person find a professional competent to deal with specific issues? Anyone who opens the yellow pages in a major metropolitan area will find page after page of therapists, ranging from marriage and family therapists to licensed social workers to licensed psychologists. What about everyone in between? As a consumer, it can be difficult to decipher all the letters after a person's name. Furthermore, those living in smaller communities or rural areas may not have more than a handful of therapists from which to choose, and there may not be anyone competent to address the issues related to DID.

Someone reading this book with the intention of finding a therapist who treats DID, however, may already have been diagnosed or suspects that she or a loved one is dissociative. Only rarely do individuals walk into therapy for the first time and announce that they have DID, but it does happen. The typical scenario is that an individual, usually female, enters therapy because of intrusive thoughts, anxiety, or depression that is interfering with her quality of life. If a diagnosis of DID or DDNOS is made, it usually occurs over time, for varied reasons. One is that the internal system that supports the dissociative process will be intact. Alters who are in place to protect the system are going to be very careful about not letting the therapist get too close initially. It usually takes weeks, or even months, for a client to trust a therapist enough to allow other parts to emerge within the therapy office. Even if switching does occur, it is very subtle at times. Often the therapist may not recognize it at first, which explains in part why individuals with DID are so easily misdiagnosed. Once the diagnosis is made, a client may very well decide to stay with her therapist, regardless of the amount of training or experience the therapist has with dissociation. If not, however, how can someone go about finding the therapist best suited to her needs?

The best approach is consumer driven. In other words, the person seeking therapy needs to decide what she is looking for and then shop until she finds the best fit. First, the individual must do her homework. If someone already knows that she has DID, she needs to find someone with expertise in that area. Best is to find someone who understands trauma disorders in general as well. A person can easily ask others for referrals without telling anyone she has DID. She might ask a doctor for a referral to a therapist who treats sexual abuse, trauma, or posttraumatic stress disorder. If she has friends who have seen therapists, she might ask them for names. Clergy often have referral lists of therapists in the community with whom they have developed relationships. Anyone a person respects and trusts is a potential referral source. The yellow pages, mental health newspapers, or women's press pages generally carry ads by therapists that sometimes list their specialty areas as well. The Internet is also a wonderful source. Just type in key words related to DID. Many search engines allow people to type in questions. For example, you might ask, "Where can I find therapists in the state of Michigan who treat DID?" Then you can continue the research from there. Those people belonging to a health maintenance organization can check their provider booklets. The ISSD, listed in appendix B, is also a good contact. Then, once three or four names have been gathered, it is time to begin narrowing down the selections to call. If a person has thought about what she is looking for, she can compose a list of initial questions to begin asking therapists.

CONTACTING THERAPISTS

A therapist usually does not have time to talk at length over the phone. Introduce yourself, explain that you are looking for a therapist, and ask if he or she has a few minutes to answer some questions. Some therapists will answer your questions over the phone, others will offer a twenty- to thirty-minute free consultation, and still others will expect you to come in for an intake session billed at the regular rate. Any of these responses is appropriate. Meeting outside of the office for coffee or lunch is never appropriate, however. If a therapist suggests getting together casually to talk, hang up and move on to the next name on the list. If a therapist refuses to answer even basic questions over the phone regarding qualifications or fees or seems offended by your desire to talk with several therapists before making a decision, consider that a red flag. A competent and professional therapist understands and encourages a client's right to make an informed decision regarding therapy. So, what might your questions be? Basic questions include the following:

Do you treat DID? If so, what is your general philosophy regarding treatment?
If you have done your research, you will probably have some ideas about what you are looking for in therapy. At the very least, you might have some ideas about what you are not looking for, which can be just as important sometimes. The most important issue in any DID treatment is empowering the client to live a more integrated life,

living with increased awareness and internal cooperation. That does not mean that parts have to disappear or cease to exist. The client makes that decision much later in therapy. It also does not mean that you have to relive every terrible memory that you carry, nor does it mean that each alter will need extensive therapy. Given those parameters, therapists will still come from different theoretical backgrounds and will use varying techniques in therapy. Those techniques are important to know before making a decision.

Are you licensed? If not, why not?

A license means that a therapist has completed the requirements set by a particular licensing board as a prerequisite for practicing. It is not a guarantee of good therapy. Typically, therapists are psychologists, clinical social workers, marriage and family therapists, or licensed professional counselors. You may occasionally find someone who is a licensed pastoral counselor. This meas clergy who have special training in counseling, or professional therapists who have received additional training in theology and have completed internships in pastoral care settings. All licensed therapists will have master's degrees, and many will have doctorates. What is most important is their levels of training and experience in treating DID or their willingness to obtain adequate training and supervision from someone who is more experienced. Many people are confused by the difference between psychologists and psychiatrists, and the distinction is important. Psychiatrists are medical doctors who specialize in psychiatry. Some psychiatrists see patients for therapy, but most deal primarily with medication issues.

Not all therapists choose to become licensed. Occasionally this is due to not being able to meet the board requirements, but in many cases it is a personal choice. Some therapists simply do not see a need for licensure or have ethical issues regarding governing boards. A lack of a license does not mean that the person is a poor therapist, but you need to use caution if dealing with an unlicensed therapist unless you know that she has the same training as her licensed counterparts and, most important, has not had a license revoked for unethical behavior. If you have any questions regarding licensure or the oversight of unlicensed professionals, do not hesitate to contact the various licensing boards in your area.

How much do you charge? Do you accept insurance? Do you offer a sliding fee scale?

Information on fees is important to have, but try to avoid making money your primary motivation in choosing a therapist if at all possible. Remember that you are making an investment in your life by entering therapy. A good investment means getting the best return on your dollar, which is why you should look for someone who has a good understanding of DID and the issues related to the disorder. It is also important to be honest regarding your own financial situation. It is difficult to have a good working relationship with someone if you are less than honest. For example, asking a therapist to lower fees when you are capable of paying the normal fee can create unnecessary resentments and affect the therapeutic relationship in a negative way.

What is your policy regarding emergencies? Am I able to reach you in the case of an emergency?

The early stages of DID therapy can be especially difficult. Although issues vary from client to client, it is certainly not unusual for emergencies to arise. Such emergencies run the gamut from suicidal thoughts to switching ego states at inappropriate times, thus creating internal chaos. The very first thing a therapist will help you to do is create safety for yourself. You need to know that someone is available twenty-four hours a day should you need help. In all likelihood, that person will not be the therapist. Therapists will, however, help you develop resources and create a safety plan. They will also need to be clear with you as to what they will and will not do in the event of an emergency. Remember that the primary goal of DID therapy is to empower the client.

What is your level of experience with treating DID?

Both training and experience are important, but regardless of the therapist's experience, you need to feel comfortable with that person. All things being equal, you will want a therapist who is experienced in treating DID as well as other related issues with which you might be dealing, such as depression or an alter who is bulimic. You also want this therapist to be someone you like and with whom you feel comfortable. If you cannot find someone like that, there is nothing wrong with seeing a less experienced therapist, provided that person is getting adequate supervision from someone who is more experienced. Once you have done your homework and have interviewed a few therapists, let your intuition aid you in making your choice.

What are your beliefs about integration?
Do you see it as a necessary goal of treatment?

There are two possible long-term goals of therapy. One is to fuse the alters so that they cease to exist as separate parts. For years, this method has been the goal of therapy with multiples. Some people, however, feel that an equally viable goal is that of co-consciousness, with each part working in cooperation with the others, much like members of a family might operate if they hope to live in any kind of harmony. Ultimately, this decision lies with the client, not the therapist. It is important, though, to discuss the pros and cons of possible outcomes with whichever therapist you choose.

How do you deal with child alters?

There are different beliefs about what is appropriate or even helpful in terms of working with younger parts. Any work that is done with alters that serves to create more separation among parts or to create unnecessary dependency on the therapist is inappropriate. Pretending that the alters do not exist, however, is equally damaging. A therapist needs to feel comfortable with dealing with child parts when they appear and must be prepared to deal with memories that may surface in these parts during sessions. Helping the client to learn how to deal effectively with child parts means that the therapist will need to interact with them as well, but the therapist also needs to be flexible enough to work with them as they are ready. That does not mean that each part will need to do her own extensive individual therapy. An adult part, typically the host (the part that has control of the body the majority of the time), will need to be present for therapy. She does not have to be present at every moment, but an adult part does need to take responsibility for the direction of therapy, getting to and from the therapist's office, and so on. Although such actions rarely flow smoothly in the beginning of therapy, this is one of its goals. In chapter 5, each stage of therapy is examined in greater detail.

A small number of therapists become surrogate parents for child alters and attempt to provide the love and nurturing that the client was denied in childhood. Although the client may crave this type of attention due to attachment issues, it is not helpful and, in fact, may be harmful. Good therapists will take a nurturing stance toward child alters, but will be very careful to keep the same boundaries with child alters that they would have with any other child client. The other extreme regarding this issue is therapists who refuse to deal with child alters at all. Their response is that clients need to learn to nurture the child parts. Although true, what these therapists are forgetting is that you may not fully understand what that means because it was not likely to be something you experienced on a consistent basis. An effective therapist can model nurturance for you without crossing boundaries and can educate you in ways of nurturing the younger parts of your self.

How do you deal with angry alters?

A DID therapist needs to be comfortable with clients expressing anger and also must be able to establish clear boundaries for the safety of both the therapist and the client. Angry parts are often protectors who keep the system safe by pushing others away. Some carry the anger of past experiences, and others are parts that have internalized characteristics of the abuser. In therapy, it is important for the client's anger to be owned and worked through. Sometimes people are afraid of their own anger and may even think it is proof that they are bad. Therapists can demonstrate stability by their presence, as they bear witness to the client's expression of her anger. Dealing with angry alters means allowing, and even encouraging, the anger to be expressed as long as it is done in a way that is not harmful. The therapist will help the client to see that anger does not have to be dangerous or always acted on. Because anger is often related to grief, the therapist will also help the client to become vulnerable enough to talk about what else lies beneath the anger.

How do you deal with memories?

A DID therapist will listen, without judgment, to the client's experience and will not attempt to determine what is or is not true. In fact, a therapist will help the client deal with the meaning attached to the memory more so than analyzing the content that is presented. If therapeutic work is done on specific memories, the client may feel as if he is reliving the memory. Good therapists do work on creating both internal and external safety for the client before delving into memory work. They also understand that it is not necessary to relive every memory and that it could actually be retraumatizing to attempt to do so. If a memory presents itself without warning in the form of a flashback, the therapist will help the client to process it, while offering grounding techniques that help the person to differentiate between then (the trauma) and now.

Recognize that there may be other questions specific to your needs or desires. How a therapist answers those questions may be helpful in your decision-making process. Once you have verified that the therapist is competent to deal with your issues, be aware that therapists operate differently. What you are looking for is compatibility. As a therapist, I have had potential clients ask for my treatment philosophy, state that they are looking for someone who is Christian, or even ask if I am available to handle emergencies twenty-four hours a day. There is not one right answer to any of these questions; it all boils down to beliefs and style. Yet it is much more profitable for both the client and the therapist if those issues are addressed up front. Although it can be time consuming to interview therapists, think of it as a learning experience. Interviewing is an excellent opportunity to learn how different therapists deal with the issues associated with DID, and also helps you feel more confident as you enter into a therapeutic relationship.

TREATMENT APPROACHES

Another issue to consider is the therapist's theoretical background and approach to treatment. There are various theoretical positions within the field of psychology, and there are many treatment approaches developed within the context of each of those theories. It would be easy to write an entire book based on the theories of psychotherapy. The focus here, however, is on the most common approaches used for the treatment of DID. I do not believe that traditional talk therapy, in and of itself, is always enough to treat DID effectively. The DID client has to make meaning out of what has happened to her. Answering the "why's" of her life, infusing them with new meaning, and learning to manage emotions in the here and now are the hallmarks of treatment for dissociative disorders. Many therapists treating DID will operate from one theoretical perspective, typically psychodynamic, and then pick and choose from other treatment options that fit the specific work they are doing. Although DID therapy addresses the past, that is not the primary focus with most therapists. The most important goal is for the client to learn to function more effectively in the here and now even while she is processing difficult material from the past. Work with alters still has to be done, but not at the expense of improving daily functioning. In other words, the client is seen as a whole person who can take responsibility for her behavior despite having to process traumatic material and regardless of the use of dissociative defenses that have resulted in the development of distinct ego states.

In the following pages, the use of cognitive therapy, psychodynamic therapy, and Adlerian therapy along with other approaches for the treatment of DID are discussed. More specific adjunct therapeutic techniques, such as eye movement desensitization reprocessing and dialectical behavior therapy, are discussed in chapter 6.

Lauren entered therapy due to a severe depression. If she were honest about it, she would have to admit that she had struggled with depression most of her life. This time was different, though. Therapy started easily enough. She walked into the psychologist's office, somewhat tentatively, and sat down. *How hard can this be?* she thought. She'd been to therapy before, as a teenager. She was depressed then, too, but it took awhile for anyone to recognize it. As a teen, she found it much easier to yell at her parents and stay out past curfew than to talk honestly about what she was feeling. Maybe she didn't even know. Now, though, as a thirty-three-year-old woman, she knew she was dealing with depression. It was getting harder and harder to even get out of bed in the mornings. With two young children, she had plenty to do during the day, but when her husband came home in the evenings she often had a difficult time even remembering what she had done all day. She also found herself looking for excuses to sit the kids in front of the television for one more viewing of *Pocahontas* or *Barney*. "I love you. You love me." The music seemed so far away. As long as it kept them entertained she was fine. She felt so exhausted that she couldn't even move.

Lauren related all this information to her therapist and patiently answered the questions about family history, previous therapy, current medications, and so on. She continued going to therapy on a weekly basis and played the dutiful patient. Six months later, though, instead of feeling better, she was getting noticeably worse. Life felt as if it was reeling out of control. Lauren described the last few weeks as surreal. "I get up every morning. I take care of my children. I attempt to take care of the house." She laughed slightly. "Yet hours go by and I do not know what I've done."

Lauren was also carrying a secret. The voices that had been conversing inside her head since childhood were getting louder. She feared she was going crazy. She wanted to quit therapy before her psychologist realized what was happening, but she was afraid she would not be able to continue to manage on her own. At least the weekly sessions provided her with some boundaries. If she could just make it from one appointment to the next without acting on the internal taunts to kill herself, maybe it would all go away.

Then, however, the diagnosis was made. Lauren had gone to her appointment as usual. She didn't look well. How could she? She was only getting four or five hours of sleep a night and was spending so much time and energy trying to block out the sound of the voices that she had little left to accomplish anything else. She sank down into the warmth and comfort of the tan couch in the therapist's office. When she felt uncomfortable during a session, she would stare at the tiny blue specks in the fabric of the couch. Today, the therapist was asking about her fifth birthday. *What is this about?* she asked herself. *Did I say something about that birthday before? Why can't this idiot just shut up?* She jumped, startled at the sound of a foreign voice. Had she actually said something? The therapist was still talking and didn't seem to be the least bit offended. The voice must have come from inside. Then it happened. "Is something wrong, Lauren?" the therapist asked.

Lauren snapped at him. "My name is Loren, and I want you to leave Lauren alone. She's tired. Leave us all alone!"

How therapy proceeds at this point depends in part on the theoretical perspective and training of the therapist.

THEORETICAL PERSPECTIVES IN TREATING DID

Therapists tend to be trained more specifically in one particular theory, even if they are versed in others as well. Although psychodynamic therapy is often employed in the treatment of DID, cognitive and Adlerian approaches are well suited for the treatment of this disorder. Following are descriptions of cognitive, psychodynamic, and Adlerian models of therapy and how they might be utilized in the treatment of DID.

Cognitive Therapy

The cognitive therapy approach is based on the work of Albert Ellis and Aaron Beck, among others. Beck's emphasis is on identifying internal beliefs and cognitive distortions. Is the client's thinking about particular issues adaptive or maladaptive? If it is maladaptive, it seems reasonable that negative emotions will follow. The basic belief is that with any situation there will be corresponding thoughts. Those thoughts will lead to feelings and eventually to actions. Of course, an important component in this reasoning is the underlying belief that we can make choices about what we think. In the case of DID, the cognitive approach is a very empowering therapy because it helps clients recognize that they have choices about how they will react to events. The cognitive therapist will intervene by helping the client become aware of cognitive distortions and create more adaptive thoughts. The therapist will use questioning in such a way as to disprove the client's own faulty logic and help her see how her own negative thoughts are affecting her life.

LAUREN: How can I expect to have any long-lasting relationships? I feel like damaged goods. Why would somebody abuse a child unless she did something to encourage it? I can't go on. I've tried to put the past out of my mind and I can't.

THERAPIST: Do you really believe that you caused the abuse?

LAUREN: (Looking down at the floor) I know it doesn't make sense, but it feels true.

THERAPIST: How old is your daughter?

LAUREN: She's six. You know that.

THERAPIST: Help me understand, then. Are you saying that if someone sexually abused your six-year-old daughter, you

would have to assume that she had done something to
encourage it?

LAUREN: Of course not!

THERAPIST: Yet in your case you expect me to believe that it
is true.

Lauren smiled and nodded, knowingly. Then the therapist stepped
up to the marker board hanging on the wall.

THERAPIST: Let's suppose, for the sake of argument, that
you did cause the abuse. How do you feel when you think
about the words, "I caused the abuse"?

LAUREN: I feel bad.

THERAPIST: Okay. What are some other words that mean
the same as bad?

LAUREN: Well, I guess I feel guilty and a little depressed
maybe.

THERAPIST: I wonder if that depression is associated with a
feeling of shame?

LAUREN: (Beginning to cry) Yes. I just cannot understand
what I could have done to encourage him.

The therapist writes down what Lauren is saying and asks her if it
looks something like this sentence: *I caused the abuse and this equals
guilt, depression, and shame.* She agreed, and he picked up a different-
colored marker and started writing again. He stepped back from
the marker board and Lauren saw that he had written new words:

I WAS AN INNOCENT CHILD WHO WAS TAKEN ADVANTAGE OF.

THERAPIST: Okay, Lauren, let's suppose this statement is
true. How does it make you feel?

LAUREN: Sad for that little girl. A little bit angry too,
   I guess. (Once again the therapist writes down what she
   was saying.) I was an innocent child who was taken
   advantage of equals sad and angry.

THERAPIST: And powerless, maybe?

LAUREN: It's weird. I'm also feeling kind of relieved.

THERAPIST: I am glad to hear that you are feeling some
   relief, too. Are you ready to do some homework?

LAUREN: (Laughing) Sure, if you promise it will make me
   feel better.

THERAPIST: This is what I want you to do. When you
   notice bothersome feelings coming up this week, chart
   them, much like we did today. Write down the situation,
   the thoughts associated with it, and the feelings that
   follow. If you are able to change the thoughts, that's great.
   If not, that's okay, too. Bring the journal to your next
   session and we will work on it together.

Rational emotive therapy is a related cognitive therapy developed
by Albert Ellis. He also addresses rational versus irrational ways of
thinking. His ABC model is a very helpful tool for assisting clients
to take control of their thoughts. In this model, A stands for the activating event, B stands for the client's beliefs about that event, and
C stands for the consequences of those beliefs, which would include,
for example, emotions and behaviors. Finally, the model includes D
for disputing irrational beliefs. The premise behind this therapy is
that people are not disturbed primarily by what happens to them,
but by their beliefs about the events in their lives. Consequently, irrational beliefs lead to negative consequences. Ellis developed a list
of core irrational beliefs. An example of one of those beliefs is that
it is awful and catastrophic when things are not the way one would

very much like them to be. Obviously, if a person truly believes something that is irrational, she will be setting herself up to be continually disappointed with self and others. The major focus in therapy is on part D of the model, disputing the irrational beliefs. This focus is extremely important in the treatment of DID because changing irrational beliefs is essential for creating cooperation and safety among internal parts.

Many therapists incorporate cognitive work into their sessions with DID clients. By offering a more realistic and empowering outlook, cognitive work is helpful for clients to use when they get caught up in negative thinking that leads down a road of powerlessness and hopelessness. Cognitive therapy teaches concrete skills that can be taken outside the therapist's office and put into practice. It also helps people take responsibility for their lives and feelings, rather than externalizing and remaining a victim even after the danger has passed.

Lauren walked into therapy looking like she had been up all night. The therapist inquired about it, and she said she did not sleep well because she was worried about something.

THERAPIST: Do you want to talk about it?

LAUREN: I guess so, but I don't really think it will do any good.

THERAPIST: What happened?

LAUREN: I was watching a movie about this woman whose husband died unexpectedly, and I started thinking that that could happen to me. I don't know what I'd do if I were alone. I couldn't even get it out of my head last night. I tried going to bed, but I couldn't sleep. Then I tried watching television, but I couldn't concentrate because of all the chatter going on in my head.

THERAPIST: Chatter?

LAUREN: Younger parts, maybe. I don't know! I get so dizzy that I can't think straight.

THERAPIST: I believe you. What do you want to do with this?

LAUREN: I want to figure out why I am so worried about it.

THERAPIST: Fair enough. Let's start there. Where would you put all this on the ABC model?

LAUREN: Well . . . (sighs), let me think for a minute. (Lauren closed her eyes and let herself sink into the couch. After a couple of minutes, she opened her eyes, took a deep breath, and started to talk.) Okay, A is for the activating event, and that means what happened, right? (The therapist nodded.) Well, I saw the movie about the woman's husband dying and it made me anxious.

THERAPIST: Okay. What happened next?

LAUREN: B is for belief. I always get confused on this one. Okay. My thoughts. I am going to be alone. My husband is going to die. I'll never be able to support myself. I don't have the energy to raise two little girls and work full-time, too.

THERAPIST: What does that say about life?

LAUREN: Life?

THERAPIST: You said I am going to be alone, but you also seem to be troubled that it could really happen. It sounds as if this belief is based on fear, not facts. So, how would you complete the sentence, Life is . . .

LAUREN: Life is out of my control and it shouldn't be! (Starts crying) I don't feel like I ever have control.

THERAPIST: Open your eyes and stay with me. When you have those thoughts, what follows?

LAUREN: Anxiety. Major anxiety.

THERAPIST: Anything else?

LAUREN: I start to feel little, like I do right now.

THERAPIST: Little? I wonder what emotion goes with being little. Powerlessness, maybe?

LAUREN: Definitely. Anxious and powerless.

THERAPIST: You also look really sad.

LAUREN: (As if she does not hear) I roam the house all night because I can't sleep.

THERAPIST: So it sounds as if this issue hinges on the belief that you are powerless. What do you think?

LAUREN: I am powerless. (She scoots to the floor and puts a blanket around herself.)

THERAPIST: I need Lauren to stay here. If you want to stay equal with this "little," you can, but I need you to come closer (Therapist motions for her to come closer) so that I can be sure that you are listening. A little bit closer still. Now, tell me about some times when you do have power. Think about now and your life as an adult.

LAUREN: Well, I know I am a good mom. Even now, when I am so tired all the time, I still try to put my kids first. My home is a lot more organized than some people's I know.

THERAPIST: Great! What else?

LAUREN: I'm good with money. I don't like taking care of the checkbook and paying bills because it is so rote, but I love managing money and figuring out how to save. I know people who make more money than we do, but they never seem to get past living month to month. I've had to get pretty creative with the money sometimes, but I've managed to do it.

THERAPIST: Wonderful! What else?

LAUREN: I guess that's about it.

THERAPIST: Do you mind if I offer a couple of observations?

LAUREN: No, go ahead.

THERAPIST: You are obviously intelligent. It comes across through your speech and the way you reason, not to mention the things that you have just shared. You also know that there are times when you are able to make choices in your life. So, you are not completely powerless. Maybe it is partially about believing you should always have power or control over your circumstances and that life will be awful if you do not.

LAUREN: (Tentatively) Sure. I guess that could be true.

THERAPIST: You are going through a difficult time, and I do not want to take that away from you. I see that we're almost out of time, but I think we have more work to do on this issue. Would you be willing to take your list of irrational beliefs and see how they apply to this situation? Then practice using the ABC format in your journal this week. What do you think?

LAUREN: I'll do it. I feel better since we've talked about it. I still feel anxious about being alone, but you're right, I am not totally powerless.

THERAPIST: Where has that little part gone?

LAUREN: She's back inside in a safe place. I'm okay.

Cognitive therapists will

- challenge the client's distorted thinking/irrational beliefs;
- help the client understand the connection among thoughts, feelings, and behavior;
- typically assign homework between sessions so that clients can practice the skills learned in therapy.

Psychodynamic Therapy

The theory behind psychodynamic therapy grew out of the original work of Sigmund Freud and has been adapted over time. It is probably the approach most widely used in the treatment of DID. Psychodynamic theory believes in the influence of the unconscious on behavior and places major importance on the functions of the ego, the self, and social relationships. This theory places more emphasis on early childhood than most other approaches and assumes that we each have an internal world affected by the past that in turn affects the present. We also carry internal representations of both self and others, and these representations profoundly affect our interactions with the world. According to this theory, the development of an integrated self begins in childhood, and a fragmented sense of self develops as a result of our needs not being met in early childhood. When that happens, a child learns to "split off" the unacceptable parts of herself. Imagine what it must be like for the child who not only is not getting needs met, but is being overtly abused as well. If splitting is a normal internal defense for a child whose needs are not being met, it becomes easier to understand how a severely traumatized child can take that a step further and unconsciously create distinct internal parts that become compartmentalized in the way they operate.

Volumes could be written on the specifics of psychodynamic theory, but what is important in this context is its relationship to the therapy of DID. One belief associated with this theory is that we all possess both good and bad impulses, and it is the ability to integrate the two that is a sign of health. Although this belief is not normally stated so directly in the early stages of DID therapy, it is suggested throughout the therapy. This concept is important for people who dissociate because the process of dissociation is about banishing the unacceptable from consciousness. To be able to recognize that we all carry what might be termed unacceptable impulses is a beginning stage for incorporating those encapsulated parts back into awareness.

During treatment, the therapist will listen to the client's story and mirror back her experiences, offering interpretations that the client can eventually turn into insights of her own. This approach is typically longer than other types of therapy and, in these days of brief therapy, is often under attack as being less effective than other types. Brief, however, does not necessarily mean better, and it is very important for clients to decide what it is they hope to achieve during therapy. To address the issues of childhood abuse and create a new sense of self will take time.

The concepts of the transference/countertransference relationship in therapy are essential to this approach. Because DID is often the product of severe neglect or trauma experienced at an early age, this issue is important. Transference refers to the client's response to the therapist (and others) based on early life experiences, and countertransference refers to the therapist's response to the client based on the therapist's own life experiences. Managing this relationship and gaining new insights from it is a transformative experience that is useful in working through the dysfunctional relationship patterns created for the client in early childhood. Taking the time to address these issues helps the client create a solid sense of self, which is extremely valuable in the long run, with lasting effects.

Lauren walked into the therapist's office and sat down. The therapist smiled at her and waited for her to begin. *I hate this silence*, Lauren thought. *Why can't she ever say something first?* She took a deep breath and said, "I don't really have anything to talk about. I'm not sure why I am here." The therapist responded with something that sounded vaguely like a *hmmm*. Lauren was starting to feel anxious. "I need to think for a minute." She closed her eyes and tried to ground herself.

"Okay," she said as she opened her eyes, "I'm ready. I've been feeling kind of depressed this week. It doesn't feel like I am making much progress."

THERAPIST: What do you think progress might look like?

LAUREN: I suppose I wouldn't be feeling this way all the time. I am so tired of feeling depressed. And I want these voices to go away. I've been in therapy for a year and I think it should be over with.

THERAPIST: It sounds like you have a lot of expectations for yourself.

LAUREN: (Angrily) I suppose.

THERAPIST: You sound angry.

LAUREN: Yeah. Why don't you do something to help me?

THERAPIST: It sounds as if you think I might have some kind of power that you don't have to take away your pain. I wonder, do you think I have answers that I am purposely keeping from you?

LAUREN: Maybe.

THERAPIST: Lauren, I promise I won't purposely keep something from you that could be helpful. I want you to be able to experience emotion without feeling so over-whelmed, but learning to do that is really a process. I wonder, could you practice letting go of your expecta-tions and just accept where you are at this moment?

LAUREN: But I don't like where I am. That's the point!

THERAPIST: Let's start there. At this moment in time, you are dealing with depression and you don't like that. What if you were to accept that, as is, rather than labeling the depression as bad and pushing it away?

LAUREN: Maybe I could, but I still don't like it.

THERAPIST: That's okay. You don't have to like it. We've

talked a lot over the past few months about how you have
pushed feelings away all your life and have let other parts
deal with them. I wonder, is the depression a way of
pushing other feelings away as well?

Lauren sat silently and stared at the floor. The therapist said
nothing at first, but then asked Lauren what was happening
inside. Lauren did not answer. The therapist thought about
whether or not she should say anything or wait for Lauren to
work through the feelings herself. Finally she said, softly,
"You are sending a clear message that you are needing something from me, but I don't know what that is. Maybe you
could start by telling me what's happening right now."
Lauren looked up slightly and then reached over and picked
up the stuffed animal sitting near her, a small brown puppy.
She held the puppy close to her chest and started to cry. "I
don't know what's happening. I just feel sad and kind of little.
There's too much noise in my head!" The therapist smiled
empathetically and nodded, asking if Lauren needed anything
from her. She shook her head no, but she looked very young
and confused, even though the therapist was looking at an
adult woman's body.

THERAPIST: We're almost out of time and I think we need
    to work on containment before you leave. I do not want
    you to drive until an adult is in charge. Is that okay with
    you? (Lauren nodded, as the tears continued to flow.)
THERAPIST: Okay, Lauren, make yourself comfortable and
    close your eyes. Imagine your safe place inside and gather
    everyone together. I can see that younger parts are out.
    Who's going to take care of the kids?
LAUREN: Lori will.

THERAPIST: Good. Let me know when the kids are tucked away safely.

Lauren watched inside her mind as three younger parts trotted off with Lori, a teenage alter who typically came out to soothe the children. Lauren had an elaborate house inside with safe rooms for everyone. Lori took the children to their playroom, where the scary feelings couldn't touch them. As the process took place, the therapist saw a change in Lauren's face, a softening. She began to breathe a bit more deeply and then settled even further into the couch.

THERAPIST: Okay, Lauren. Notice whether anyone else is needing anything.

Lauren continued to sink into the couch. Her breath was deep and rhythmic. After a few minutes she opened her eyes. The two sat in silence for a minute, and then the therapist asked how she was doing. Lauren nodded and said that she was okay. She looked and felt exhausted from the entire process.

LAUREN: I think I'm going to walk around for a few minutes before I drive home.
THERAPIST: That sounds like a good idea. It is good to see you are doing things to take care of yourself. We already have a time set for next week, but you can always call and leave a message if you are feeling a need to check in before then.

With that, Lauren left the session, knowing that the work of learning to connect with her feelings was going to be a major undertaking. She hoped she was ready.

Psychodynamic therapists will

- interpret what the client shares;
- assist clients in working through the transference relationship;
- help to bring disowned parts of the self into awareness.

Adlerian Therapy

Adlerian theory is sometimes categorized as a cognitive therapy and sometimes as a psychodynamic therapy because it contains essential elements of both. Alfred Adler was originally a contemporary of Freud, but they parted company due to disagreements regarding certain aspects of Freudian theory. Adler believed that each individual is unique and develops a lifestyle from which goals and resulting behaviors are derived. The basic principles of Adlerian psychology include the following:

1. We are social beings who want to belong.
2. We are self-determining and creative individuals who possess the power for change.
3. We are goal directed, and our behaviors have a purpose.
4. Life is subjective. We are the ones who give it meaning.
5. It is important to view both self and others from a holistic perspective.

Other components of Adlerian psychology are equally well suited to the treatment of DID. They include a belief in respect for each individual, equality between client and therapist, and continuous encouragement for the client as she begins to address her abuse issues and the ways those experiences have shaped her current reality. Of course, the way it plays out in therapy depends partially on the therapist's style and personality, not to mention the way the therapist/client relationship unfolds.

Respect and equality can be played out in a number of ways. The most basic is in attitude. Adlerian-trained therapists try to see each client as a unique individual who is worthy of a happy and productive life. Thus, they consciously have to work at keeping unburdened prejudices and judgments out of the therapeutic relationship. Adlerian therapists want to be able to see the client and themselves as two people who are walking a path together. When treatment plans are written or new therapy techniques are employed, they will discuss them with the client, explain their rationale, and ask for the client's input. Then they will decide together on the direction the therapy will go. If the client feels uncomfortable with something that is happening, the therapist wants her to feel comfortable enough to tell, and if therapy is doing something that is not helpful, the therapist wants her to be able to say no.

The encouragement piece for an Adlerian therapist is important as well. In the case of DID, encouragement might take the form of cheerleading when progress is made at practicing self-soothing during a time of emotional distress. It might manifest as nurturance when a client is feeling hopeless. It is like the "good parent" who says to the child, "You can do it. I believe in you."

One important Adlerian principle that relates directly to DID is the belief that we each possess a drive to feel significant. Is it not true that we all want to feel a sense of mastery or purpose in our lives? We carry with us a self-concept or view of ourselves "as is." We also carry a self-ideal; the view of our self as we believe it ought to be. Then we place that view of self into our carefully molded view of the world, which includes our general beliefs about other people and the way the world operates coupled with our own ethical convictions. Put it all together and you have a working model of your lifestyle, or a psychological map. According to Adler, you will then be in the business of seeking mastery in the various life tasks: social, work, and love. We each set about life on our search for significance, much like a prospector in search of gold. What is so reassuring about it is that we are on the journey together, with the knowledge that there is enough significance to go around. If I experience mastery on a life task, it does not take away from your ability to experience mastery as well. This theory actually suggests that it is normal for humans to have problems and that the search for perfection is abnormal.

The Adlerian belief in the courage to be imperfect allows us to rest in the knowledge that we can be "good enough" and that we can afford our fellow travelers on life's path the same. The goal for the dissociative person is the same as for anyone else: a sense of mastery and significance in life. The battle lies in the tendency to fall into discouragement and to lose the courage for facing life. When that happens, the energy for living is poured into protecting the self. In childhood, when a person is facing abuse or other trauma, that response actually makes sense. In adulthood, however, once the trauma has passed, the energy directed toward survival needs to be poured into living as a person who wants to experience a more satisfying life. That is a major outcome of therapy.

The basic principles of Adlerian therapy, coupled with these important concepts, provide a stable framework for successful therapy to emerge. The Adlerian therapist will also address the concept of mistaken beliefs in much the same way as a cognitive therapist would. Adler believed that the healthiest people are the ones who are able to look beyond their own suffering to see and respond to the suffering of others in an empathic way. He referred to this belief as social interest. In the case of DID, social interest begins at home. It is imperative for alter personalities to learn to cooperate if healing is to occur. Cooperation, however, cannot be sustained over time if there is no mutual respect among internal parts. This respect will develop over time through therapist modeling, treatment interventions, and the therapeutic relationship itself. As this cooperative effort begins to take shape among parts and as the client becomes healthier, she can eventually begin to express social interest outside the system as well. As therapists, Adlerians can embrace the belief in social interest by extending their own concerns to a population that has struggled to survive in a world that has offered them little reason to believe in their fellow human beings.

Lauren plopped down on the therapist's couch and started talking about how Mari's (a teen part) bulimia was creating too many problems for her.

LAUREN: I can't get anything done. I'll start eating and then I blank out. Sometimes I come to while I'm bent over the toilet puking my guts out. Other times I "wake up" and two or three hours have passed and the kitchen's a wreck and I'm exhausted. I know it is Mari, but I sure as hell don't know what to do about it!

THERAPIST: Let's remember that Mari is a part of you. I think it will be helpful to take that approach in the long run. Do you know what's causing this binge/purge behavior?

LAUREN: I think so, but I'm not positive.

THERAPIST: How can you find out?

LAUREN: (Smiling sheepishly) Ask?

THERAPIST: Okay. Why don't you check in with Mari right now? If she needs to talk, that's fine, but you can talk for her if you like. Take a deep breath and take as much time as you need.

Lauren took a deep breath and closed her eyes. She could sense Mari's presence inside and explained that they needed to work on the eating disorder issue together. Mari agreed and began to answer Lauren's questions. This internal conversation all happened while the therapist sat waiting patiently. Lauren's internal system had created a meeting room inside where conversations such as this one could take place. Once she and Mari had connected and exchanged information, Lauren returned her consciousness to the therapy office. She opened her eyes and blinked a few times. The therapist had learned that the blinking was a sign that either internal communication or switching among parts was taking place.

Lauren was the host and was easily recognized, but something was different now. She looked hard and very intense.

MARI: I binge so that she won't get so fucking freaked out by feelings. Then she panics anyway and I purge to get rid of it. She's so stupid!

THERAPIST: You really work hard to protect her, don't you?

MARI: What's that supposed to mean?

THERAPIST: It sounds as if you believe feelings are dangerous or too much for Lauren to handle.

MARI: Definitely too much. It doesn't take much to overwhelm her. Without me she would have been dead a long time ago.

THERAPIST: Would you be willing to try a little experiment?

MARI: That depends on what it is.

The therapist picked up a pad that was lying on the table next to her. She began to write, then tore off a sheet and handed it to Mari. Mari read it and laughed. The note was short and to the point. It said, "Rx: Start acting 'as if' Lauren can handle feelings. Report back in one week."

MARI: Okay, but it won't work.

THERAPIST: If you are willing to try, that's good enough for
    me. By the way, have you ever thought about how life
    would be different without the symptom use?

MARI: Well, I'd have to start dealing with feelings, I mean
    she would, and that's scary. She is *sooo* pathetic! We'd also
    have more time to do fun things, though, and that's good.

THERAPIST: (Laughing) True! More time is always good.

MARI: Do you think I'm bad because I binge and purge?

THERAPIST: Not at all. I think you have been working hard
    to protect everyone inside. Maybe it's time to take a rest.

MARI: If I go inside, can I come back sometime if I want to?

THERAPIST: Absolutely!

At that, Mari closed her eyes, as if in a trance. Soon
Lauren opened her eyes, looking somewhat disconnected for
a moment. The therapist asked what she had been aware of
while Mari was out. Then, when Lauren felt more grounded,
they ended the session.

Adlerian therapists will

- address a client's misbeliefs;
- assess a client's lifestyle;
- typically assign homework that challenges the client to
  behave in new ways.

OTHER PERSPECTIVES

In many ways, cognitive, psychodynamic, and Adlerian therapies are
similar, yet in other ways, they are very different. Although none was

developed specifically for treating DID, each has something to offer. Many other theoretical perspectives are being incorporated into work with DID clients, including feminist therapy, family systems theory, ego-state therapy, and object relations theory, to name a few. We now take a brief look at each of these.

Feminist Therapy

Feminist therapy is about empowering women and validating their strengths as opposed to pathologizing their experiences with labels such as dependent and hysterical. It is also about helping individual women find their voices rather than automatically adopting the societal roles assigned to them. It is not about empowering women at the expense of men, which would only serve to create deeper societal wounds, nor is it about promoting a political agenda.

Feminist therapy builds on client strengths, is supportive and nonblaming, and focuses on the ways in which society influences beliefs and behavior. Foremost, it stresses the importance of individual choices and responsibility for all people. In the treatment of DID, feminist approaches to therapy can help clients to focus on personal strengths and the development of a greater sense of self. It can also help clients begin to make sense of past experience by exploring it within a cultural, as well as a personal, context.

Family Systems Theory

The traditional approach to family systems therapy views the family as a unit (system) in which each member is affected by the others and in which the system as a whole is affected by the individual. Consequently, behavior changes in one person will affect the balance of the entire system. The primary tenets of family systems therapy have been adapted into an internal family system (IFS) approach that can be useful when thinking about DID.[1]

In the IFS approach, it is believed that it is the nature of the mind to be subdivided into "parts." DID is simply a more extreme manifestation of this concept. According to this model, there are no "bad" parts; as we develop, our parts develop too. The overall goals of IFS therapy are to achieve balance and harmony within the internal system and to increase positive and purposeful communication among the self and other parts (subpersonalities).

Ego-State Therapy

Ego-state therapy is a psychodynamic approach that is integrated with traditional psychodynamic theory and often directed through hypnosis. Ego-state therapy, developed by John Watkins and Helen Watkins, uses group and family therapy techniques to resolve conflicts among various "ego states." This concept is especially important when working with dissociation because the "parts" experienced by someone with DID are similar to the "ego states" common to all persons. They are simply more distinct and overt in multiplicity.[2]

Working with ego states is much like working with an internal family that makes up what we call *the Self*. According to John Watkins, an ego state may be defined as an organized system of behavior and experiences the elements of which are bound together by some common principle. The use of ego-state therapy helps bring about increased awareness and communication among internal parts in a dissociated system.[3]

Object Relations Theory

Practitioners of object relations theory, an aspect of psychodynamic theory, believe that relationships are primary and are foundational to the development of an identity, or a Self. Because DID is primarily a disturbance in identity, it makes sense in therapy to explore early relationships. The initial focus would be the mother/infant (or other primary caregiver) relationship. Yet it is not simply the relationship, but *how* primary relationships are perceived and internalized by the client that are important. These experiences are believed to be reflected in the way the person behaves in current relationships. The "object" in object relations theory is the internalized image we carry within of primary relational figures, including ourselves. In DID therapy, exploring these internalized images, within the context of tradiional psychodynamic therapy, leads to a more unified sense of Self.

SUMMARY

Although there are guidelines for the effective treatment of DID, individual therapists will gravitate toward specific theories and styles of therapy. Each approach mentioned in this chapter has positive aspects to bring to treatment, but each also has common pitfalls that can occur. Briefly, the pitfalls of the primary theories include the following:

Cognitive Therapy

- Allowing the therapy to rely too much on formula as opposed to relationship.
- Becoming directive in a condescending or authoritative manner.
- Failing to approach child alters at their level of reasoning.

Psychodynamic Therapy

- The possibility of moving into trauma work before adequately addressing stabilization.
- The possibility of a therapist taking an overly intellectual or authoritarian stance in which the therapist is seen as the expert.
- Creating unnecessary distance in the relationship based on an extreme adherence to the belief that therapists should not self-disclose. This pitfall is especially problematic when working with younger alters who may interpret this behavior as a lack of caring on the part of the therapist.

Adlerian Therapy

- Taking the values of cooperation and equality to an extreme, resulting in a lack of boundaries.
- Using the concept of individual wholeness as a refusal to acknowledge the client's experience of having internal parts.
- The possibility of missing the presence of serious pathology based on the belief that labeling of any kind is detrimental to the client.

Because therapists are human, they will, of course, make mistakes. This humanity is part of what constitutes a genuine relationship. Bad therapy, however, is about consistent or intentional choices made by the therapist that are inappropriate or harmful to the client. It is important for clients to be aware of behavior that may constitute bad therapy so that they are in a better position to be good consumers. Inappropriate behavior on the part of a therapist includes poor boundaries that are manifested by personal relationships with clients outside the therapy office or by excessive self-disclosure on the part of the therapist. Any sexual contact between a therapist and a client is an extreme form of boundary violation. If this type of behavior occurs within the context of therapy, the client should immediately terminate the relationship and report the therapist's behavior to the appropriate licensing board. Another unhelpful quality that might be experienced in therapists is a rigidity about the final outcome for the therapy. With dissociative clients, such rigidity might manifest as an insistence that a final fusion among internal parts is necessary, regardless of the client's beliefs about integration. Using techniques with which a client does not feel comfortable, against her will, is also inappropriate and serves only to create distrust and an increase in internal anxiety, as does extensive focusing on child alters or trauma work before addressing stabilization issues. Shaming or blaming a client about her dissociative defenses or perceived lack of progress is not only inappropriate but can also become a reenactment of past trauma.

Finally, poor therapy is often disguised as a sloppy form of eclecticism. Eclectic therapy is therapy based on a particular theoretical perspective that is enhanced by integrating aspects of other theories when appropriate to the particular client or issue at hand. This therapy can be a very helpful and creative approach. Sloppy eclecticism, on the other hand, is when a therapist borrows from many different approaches without having a clear basis for doing so. It is always appropriate for clients to ask why a therapist is using a particular approach or to express concerns if a particular approach does not appear to be helpful.

One mistake some clients make is to think that therapist confrontation or the experiencing of uncomfortable or negative feelings constitutes bad therapy. If such a situation occurs in an abusive context, it does. Therapy, however, is not about giving advice or making people feel good; it is about the client learning to live life in a more functional way and it often involves experiencing painful feelings.

For some people, it is about learning to feel for the first time. Sometimes, therapists have to share observations or insights with a client that the client may not really want to hear, but that is part of what constitutes good therapy. Generally speaking, the quality of the relationship between the client and therapist is more important than the specific theory to which the therapist adheres, in terms of final outcome and therapy satisfaction.

Several therapist qualities can benefit the client/therapist relationship. John Watkins mentions nurturance and resonance as being important. He also mentions the ability to think like a child as being helpful in facilitating positive outcomes with child ego states.[4] Another aid to working with internal parts is flexibility, as well as the ability to adapt to whatever internal experience is being presented by the client. Other key therapist traits include empathy and respect for the client and a belief in the equality of the therapist and client, despite their differing roles. Vital to the therapeutic relationship is the creation of a secure frame that allows the client to feel safe within the context of the relationship. These characteristics certainly help create this frame, but therapist integrity and genuineness are the key ingredients in forming this foundational frame. These traits help the client feel secure in the knowledge that the therapist is trustworthy, consistent, and reliable, which creates a safe space for the client to begin to explore difficult and often painful issues.

Clients have the right to expect good therapy and to work with a therapist who is willing to discuss these issues as they arise. If you are currently looking for a therapist, consider using the form given in Figure 4.1 as a way of recording the information obtained during your interviewing process. Once you have taken that step, it can be helpful to know what to expect as the therapy process begins. In the next chapter, we look at the typical stages of therapy when treating DID.

1. Do you treat DID? Circle Yes or No
   If so, what is your general philosophy regarding treatment?
   (List key points on a separate sheet.)
2. Are you licensed? Circle Yes or No
   If not, why not? (List key points on a separate sheet.)
3. How much do you charge?
   Do you accept insurance? Circle Yes or No
   Do you accept (name of own insurance company)? Circle Yes or No
   Do you offer a sliding fee scale? Circle Yes or No
   (If yes, list the information regarding fees on a separate sheet.)
4. What is your policy regarding emergencies?
   Am I able to reach you in the case of an emergency? Circle Yes or No
   (If no, ask what other provisions are made for emergencies and list
   them on a separate sheet.)
5. What is your level of expertise in treating DID?
6. What are your beliefs regarding integration?
   Do you see integration as a necessary goal of treatment?
   Circle Yes or No
7. How do you deal with child alters? (List answers separately.)
8. How do you deal with angry alters? (List answers separately.)
9. How do you deal with memories? (List answers separately.)

Summary:
Things I think would be positive working with this therapist include:
   1.
   2.
   3.
   4.
   5.
Things I think could be unhelpful working with this therapist include:
   1.
   2.
   3.
   4.
   5.

Figure 4.1 Therapist Interview Form

Chapter Five

Stages of Therapy and What to Expect

Sarah goes to therapy, plops down on the floor, and lays out several note cards in a way she hopes will help the therapist understand how her internal "system" operates.

Mark tells the therapist he is ready to discuss a memory that he has kept to himself for twenty years. They talk about how he will create a "safe place" for himself inside as he begins to share information and feelings about the traumatic events he experienced as a child.

Kim announces that her "kids" are ready to integrate (a term DID patients often use to describe a joining together of their internal parts). She wants to create a ritual that she and her therapist can use to help celebrate this transition together.

These individuals are each engaged in a different aspect of DID therapy. In general, therapists experienced in the treatment of DID agree on the various stages necessary for treatment. These stages include some form of stabilization, trauma work, integration, and postintegration therapy. Stabilization is what occurs first. A client may or may not enter therapy with the belief that she has DID. The purpose of the internal system is to keep the disorder outside the host's consciousness, thus protecting the integrity of the system. Something, however, brings the client to therapy and that "something" is often severe depression associated with a recent crisis in the person's life. The external circumstances might not even appear to be that serious to others, but to the client, it is the external circumstances that set off the internal chaos.

Imagine going for a walk in the woods with a friend on a crisp autumn day. Your friend Paula is dissociative, but neither of you knows it. Paula was raped in a wooded area when she was a child, an event she does not clearly remember. As you walk together, you talk and laugh about the new things your kids are learning and the latest gossip around the office water cooler. Then Paula starts trembling slightly. You see the look of terror on her face and ask what's wrong. Instead of answering, though, she slowly begins to fall to the ground and then throws her arms over her head as if to shield herself. You do not know what's happening and your own anxiety starts to rise as you try to console her, but she reacts as if you are not even there. Then she looks up, startled, and asks what just happened. You explain what you saw. At first she looks confused, but then she begins to make excuses, probably more from embarrassment than anything, as you put your arms around each other and head back for the car.

Consider how frightening that would be for both of you. What Paula does not yet fully understand is that she was triggered by past memories during that walk in the woods. There was something about the way the sun was shining through the autumn leaves, coupled with the faint smell of smoke in the distance, that reminded her of the rape experience so many years ago. She reacted as if she were reliving the past without consciously remembering that particular incident. You drop her off at home with the sincere invitation to call if she needs to do so. Paula walks into the house, feeling somewhat dazed, as she tries to put the events of the day out of her mind. She makes herself a cup of tea, puts in her favorite video, and wraps up in the black and white down comforter that always makes her feel safe and warm. As the days go on, however, Paula begins to fall into a depression. She begins to experience frightening nightmares that wake her from sleep, and she doesn't know why. It is at this point that she decides to enter therapy.

STABILIZATION

As discussed in chapter 3, therapy will begin with an initial interview and the task of finding the appropriate diagnosis. A therapist might initially diagnose Paula with depression, if that is what is being presented. Eventually, though, as he interacts with her and gains more information, through verbal interaction, observation, and the emergence of various ego states, he will make the diagnosis of DID. For both the client and the therapist, that changes everything. Therapy with a DID client always begins by focusing on stabilization. The client may have entered therapy due to a crisis situation and is in need of coping techniques, but even if that is not the case, the diagnosis itself may create a kind of crisis internally. The formation of DID occurs in childhood when more primitive defenses such as splitting and dissociation are the primary means of coping. Yet the host, who is likely to be the person presenting for therapy, has probably lived her life unaware of the dissociative disorder. She will certainly be aware of the primary symptoms that are creating difficulty for her, but dissociative amnesia will cause her to be unaware of certain behaviors. The purpose of the internal system, after all, is to create safety for the mind and body. What many people would label dysfunction is actually quite adaptive given the circumstances of the DID person's life. Now, though, in the confines of a therapist's office, a client is being told that she has DID and that this disorder is the explanation for the years of distress she has been experiencing. A therapist should not be fooled into thinking that because he is feeling positive about discovering the diagnosis the client will share in his joy. For some clients, the diagnosis brings relief because it offers an explanation for the various symptoms they have been living with throughout their lives. For others, this information is difficult to digest. In fact, for some clients, having the diagnosis actually helps create a new set of problems.

ISSUES RELATED TO SELF

Who am I now that I have this diagnosis? Does this diagnosis mean I am crazy? How does my therapist know the diagnosis is accurate?

Internal Stress

Now the secret that has been kept for so many years is out in the open. As with any system, change brings stress to the overall system.

Therapeutic Relationship

How do I know I can trust my therapist? Does she have some vested interest in giving me this diagnosis?

Therapists will want to use this adjustment period as a time to educate the client about DID and its form and function. This point is also a time for discussing philosophical issues of importance to the client as she wrestles with acceptance of the diagnosis. Of course, inherent in acceptance of the diagnosis is an acceptance of past trauma or issues related to disordered attachment. DID does not develop in a vacuum. If an individual has been able to encapsulate unacceptable memory and feeling and place it outside of consciousness for so many years, the idea of past trauma might seem unbelievable. One of the hallmark comments heard from DID clients is "I don't want to lie about what happened. That would be worse than anything." A therapist's goal is not about proving whether a memory is true. Most of the time that is not even possible. Instead, therapists educate their DID clients about how memory operates and explain to them that no one's memory is 100 percent accurate. Then the therapist will talk about managing symptoms in the here and now so that life can be lived to its fullest. That means a willingness to wrestle with a lot of uncertainty. Although this stage of treatment can sometimes seem painstakingly slow to a therapist, psychoeducational and existential questions are important aspects of the client's work. Without it, the client will not develop an acceptance of the diagnosis, and without that, she will not be able to work directly on the issues related to the disorder.

Creating Safety

Other issues related to stabilization include creating a secure treatment frame, managing extreme levels of stress, creating personal safety if there is suicidal ideation or other self-injurious behaviors, and helping the client learn to recognize and manage dissociation to a limited degree. During this stage, it is important to develop a crisis plan, including a no-suicide contract. Many clinics have standard crisis plans that detail whom to call after hours if the primary therapist is not available. Crisis plans for dissociative clients, however, are much more effective if they are individualized. Many DID clients have been through previous therapy, and some have been a part of the broader mental health system. In those cases, the client will already be familiar with crisis plans and may not have a lot of faith in them. With the proper diagnosis and a therapist who is willing to work with a client in developing a plan, however, the human response can be calming in and of itself. It also sends a clear message to internal "parts" that their desires and needs are being validated. An example of a crisis plan is shown in Figure 5.1.

It is also important for therapists to help the client find a psychiatrist who believes in DID and is willing to work with the therapist in terms of hospitalization, if necessary, to ensure the client's safety. Sometimes antidepressants or antianxiety medications are helpful

---

If I, (name of client), experience emotions that feel overwhelming, I will use the coping skills that I've discussed with my therapist, including:

1. Mindful breathing

2. Writing in a journal

3. Exercising

4. Listening to music

5. Coloring or drawing

6. Conducting an internal roll call to see what parts are present and what each is feeling and needing

I agree not to use any chemicals (other than prescribed drugs used appropriately) as a way of managing symptoms. Instead, I will remind myself that "feelings cannot hurt me" and I will do at least one self-nurturing activity.

I, (name of client), agree to contact (name of therapist) if I believe I am going to hurt myself or others (internal or external). If my therapist is not available, I will contact (friend 1), (friend 2), or (area crisis line).

Figure 5.1 Sample Crisis Plan for a DID Client

in terms of stabilization as well, but medications are much more effective if the doctor truly understands the dynamics associated with DID. In addition to creating a team of health professionals, this stage is also a time for creating an overall support network. A support network includes friends, supportive family members, and possibly clergy or other spiritual support people, such as twelve-step sponsors. In addition, the client may want to include community support such as drop-in centers or support groups that are geared toward working with dissociation. The importance of establishing this network is to help the client begin to feel connected to others in a healthy way and to learn that it is acceptable to ask for help. It is also important for the therapist to acknowledge that she cannot be the sole support for her DID clients. If she tries to be, she will quickly burn out and may find herself becoming part of the problem.

Normalizing

Normalizing is an integral part of the stabilization process. The reason is twofold.

First, the client probably operates from an extremely shame-based perspective. People operating from this perspective see themselves as being defective and then make judgments about life based on that belief. Shame causes a person to want to hide for fear of being "found out" and negatively judged by others. Dissociative clients often talk about wanting to disappear and even rely on dissociation as a way to disappear and avoid further shame. Self-injury and wanting to die are the most extreme expressions of internal feelings of shame. Because shame is so central to the dissociator's belief system, it becomes important for the therapist to reeducate the client regarding traumatic stress so that she can begin to accept her own responses to the trauma that has been experienced rather than integrate it into an already formed shame-based foundation.

Second, normalization is a means of giving persons permission to tell their stories. As long as the experience is clouded in shame, it will remain hidden, but normalizing is like being reborn. What is left is the real self, albeit wounded, that was previously buried in the muck and mire of shame and guilt, but is now coming alive to new possibilities. Each opportunity for normalizing builds on the last. What is surprising to some therapists and friends is that the dissociator truly believes she is different from others regardless of how normal her life might appear. Part of that perception has to do with her carrying a secret. Many clients keep their diagnoses to themselves because they fear rejection from others if the truth were known.

Developmental issues are another reason for this belief. Because internal "parts" operate so separately from one another, the DID person really does feel five years old at times. The successful attorney with DID really might "wake up" in an unsavory bar, in a nearby city she rarely visits. Because this scenario is not typical for most of us, the belief "I am different" is reinforced. The belief is based on a shame-based identity: "I am carrying a secret. Maybe you cannot see it, but I know that it is there."

In reality, all people have issues that they are dealing with in life, and most of us are carrying secrets of one kind or another, even though they may be small. We all think, say, and do things we would rather forget. In addition, everyone has experienced the pain of rejection and failures along the way. Negative experiences and impulses are one side of being human. The more psychologically integrated a person is, the more successful that person will be at navigating rough waters. We are all at various stages of integration or psychological maturity. DID is simply the most extreme form of disintegration. Because internal parts will correspond with various levels of development ranging from childhood to adulthood, persons with DID (or individual parts, at least) may lack some of the sophisticated skills required for dealing with relationships and managing emotions. Those skills, however, can be taught, which is part of what therapy is about. Clients need to understand that all people deal with anger, depression, and loneliness, and all people deal with anxiety about various circumstances in life. The anxieties just happen to take on different forms depending on the person. For the dissociator, the importance of learning this fact is to be able eventually to reach the "Aha!" type of realization that it is not so much "I am different" as it is "I am the same. I am a part of an exclusive club that is called the human race."

Negative Beliefs

Another important element of stabilization is to address the negative cognitive framework from which the client is operating. Abuse or any other severe trauma that occurs at a young age changes the way in which a child views the world. We appear to enter the world with the innate expectation that it is a safe place and that we can expect our needs to be met. Early trauma, however, teaches us just the opposite: "The world is a dangerous place and I cannot trust others to provide me with what I need. Therefore, there must be something wrong with me. I am bad!"

It is vital for therapists to understand this underlying framework of thought because, despite the beautiful package that the client may be presenting, he is probably dealing with enormous internal conflicts that the therapist does not see. Internal parts who feel a need to protect themselves, or each other, may do their dead-level best to convince the therapist that they really are bad. Not only will that keep the cognitive framework intact, but it will also keep the therapist from getting too close. If a therapist knows what to expect, however, she can react differently than she might if caught off guard. Knowing what to expect allows for the possibility of welcoming whatever parts are experiencing the conflict so that they can begin to understand and accept the roles they have been playing to protect the system over the years. Then the therapist will normalize the behavior as much as possible.

Developing Awareness

During the stabilization stage, the client and therapist will also get to know the internal system better. Some clients will want to illustrate the system in a way that is meaningful to them, which gives the therapist much insight into the client's overall personality structure. Some clients may make elaborate flowcharts. Some may use note cards to record relevant information about each alter, a sort of minibiography. Others may illustrate the system using various shapes and colors. Some might write a story to explain life on the "inside." And, of course, some may feel powerless to do anything without the help of the therapist each step along the way. The purpose of illustrating the system is to increase awareness and further increase stability. If a therapist jumps into trauma work before gaining a general understanding of the client's internal system, it can help to create much unnecessary chaos and pain.

Awareness, however, develops differently for different people. Some clients choose to do structured activities such as the ones above. Others find that their awareness naturally increases over time as they talk about their issues in therapy. Still others find that their internal systems are so fluid and ever changing that it does not make sense to try to chart them in a formal way. Yet awareness is still important and is the first step toward developing communication among the various parts. This skill is important for the client to have so that negotiation can begin to take place in terms of what parts present for therapy, deciding how needs will be met, and negotiating safety for the entire system.

> I talk with child alters, but I do not go in search of them. I will ask what the child alter needs and help my clients provide that for these alters. When I believe that a child alter is present, I will speak with the alter, but I also request that everyone else be present and listen to what is being said. I also emphasize repeatedly that the child alters are a part of the whole person. I do not want to encourage any more splitting than what has already occurred.
>
> (Judith, therapist, Canada)

Although the components of the stabilization stage of therapy are quite straightforward, do not assume for even a second that this means it is easy. Stabilization may take up to a year or more, depending on the client. If the client is unwilling to accept the diagnosis fully, it is highly unlikely she will be able to plunge right into communication among parts. More likely is that she will approach the system work and then run when faced with internal parts (experiences, thoughts, and feelings) that she does not want to accept as an aspect of herself, or she will work on internal issues until faced with an external circumstance that feels threatening in some way. When either situation happens, she will immediately begin to employ the old survival defenses, including dissociation. Whether you are the therapist or the client, do not become disheartened. Even backward steps are a part of stabilization. The client knows precisely how fast she can go. The therapist's job is to continue to challenge damaging beliefs, to continue to aid the client in building both internal and external support, to communicate with parts, to encourage increased internal communication, and, when possible, to normalize what appears to be quite abnormal to the person experiencing it.

The interesting thing about the stages of therapy is that they are each distinct, yet fluid. Completing the stabilization stage does not mean that you will never go back to working on stabilization issues again. This fluidity will help in times of discouragement for both the therapist and client. In fact, the bulk of therapy time is spent in stabilization because it is the foundation for the rest of the treatment process. As you move from this stage you will begin the trauma work. The techniques used in processing trauma are all initially introduced and practiced in the stabilization stage, which enables clients to focus on the here and now and manage strong emotional content. Then, as trauma work becomes more focused, these techniques are reinforced.

TRAUMA WORK

Trauma work generally begins with the client's story about her abuse experience. The story might be told verbally or in written form. If the client carries high anxiety about needing to have her story told, it is sometimes told over the course of a few sessions. The story is never told just once, however. As various ego states emerge, they too will carry pieces of the story. This telling, in and of itself, is part of the trauma work because what one part says may contradict the experience of another. Continuing to educate the client about dissociation and memory is an important part of working through these internal conflicts. Internal parts may also carry information that is upsetting to others, especially the host. Feelings associated with any new information presented need to be processed as well. Integration of internal memory is a process that occurs over time as pieces of information are shared among alters and processed.

I encourage host-alter communication as the host can
tolerate it. Early in the work, alters have information that may
be useful to treatment, but that the host cannot tolerate.
I generally summarize discussions with alters to the host if
co-consciousness is not achieved yet, because secrets block
communication. Treatment is about opening communication.
  (Sandra, therapist, North Carolina)

Processing Memories

The aspect of trauma work that is generally most troublesome for
clients is the processing of memories. The reexperiencing of traumatic events is often accompanied by the emotions associated with
the event. The purpose of the memory work is to bring dissociated
material into consciousness so that the client is able to function in an
integrated manner. In therapy, this work can occur through planned
sessions in which the goal is discussed beforehand and the containment techniques learned in stage one can be reinforced. What is
most frightening for dissociators are the unplanned flashbacks that
occur when a memory is triggered, either consciously or not. Flashbacks are accompanied by floods of emotion and often involve
switching or dissociation that is experienced as extremely distressing. It is important to plan as much as possible for these sessions by
implementing coping plans and support systems and by continuing
to increase the internal communication process initially established
in stage one so that the dissociator can be helped as much as possible to differentiate between then and now.

An important issue to consider in memory work is that it not become so overwhelming for the client that she becomes retraumatized. In addition, there may be several ego states involved in one
aspect of memory work. Each of those parts, either alone or in

groupings, needs to be included in the work so as to process it most effectively. It is important to plan this work, when possible, so that small pieces of the trauma are dealt with at any given time. Such planning will allow for containment of emotions so that the client is able to work with difficult material without giving up a sense of internal safety.

Although clients need to operate within the framework of their own systems, therapists can use certain techniques to facilitate communication and contain emotions. They include watching a memory on an internal movie screen, setting up an internal video room where a memory can be played on a videotape, or having internal parts meet together around a conference room table.[1] These fairly standard techniques that therapists teach to clients not only increase internal communication, but also manage the emotions associated with spontaneous flashbacks. Both the movie screen and video room allow clients to distance themselves from the memory and feel that they have more control over the emotions associated with the memory.

When working with memories, therapists often have a client imagine a video room that meets her every need, from the comfort of the furniture to the style and size of the television. When the room is exactly as she wants it to be, the client is asked to play a video of the memory being worked on. She knows that at any time she can mute the sound, speed up the tape, pause the tape, and so on. Processing is practiced in this way so that the client begins to feel some mastery over the memory. Then, with practice, she can use this technique on her own when faced with intrusive thoughts and disturbing pictures that are associated with past trauma. A variation of this technique is to use a split-screen television on which the client can watch the memory on one side and the present time (post-trauma) on the other. Again, a remote control is used to manipulate the memory as needed. With each of these techniques, after viewing the memory, the client is asked to label the videotape and then put it away in a safe place to be taken out at a later time, if needed. This safety step is important, and clients will often choose a safe or a cabinet that only they can open.

When working with internal communication, it is helpful for clients to check in daily whether they think they need to or not. Sometimes this check-in can be a very informal roll call where someone (often the host) calls out each part's name and asks if that part has anything to share with the rest of the system. At other times, it may be more productive to have a group meeting. Some people have a specific place inside where parts of the self congregate to discuss issues that arise. If not, they can meet around a conference room table to hold a meeting. It is preferable that different parts take turns chairing the meetings and that anyone be free to call a meeting if there is an issue she wants to discuss. These guidelines allow for increased cooperation and respect among parts. Then, whoever is chairing the meeting or taking roll will pay particular attention to who enters the room, with each part being given the opportunity to participate in the discussion. Some clients find it helpful to have a microphone on the table so that each part is able to talk in turn, helping to decrease the amount of internal distraction. The technique itself is not as important as its workability for the client. Therapists can teach the basic framework and assist clients in learning containment and communication skills, but it is up to the client to adapt the techniques to her specific needs.

In the early stages of therapy, flashbacks can be perceived as mini-crises to be addressed. As coping skills are learned and internal communication is increased, however, these experiences will begin to be integrated into the client's conscious mind. As that happens, flashbacks begin to occur less frequently and with less intensity. The reexperiencing of traumatic events, however, is not enough for healing to occur. As memories are integrated, the client will be trying to make sense of the experience as well. Thus, the trauma stage of therapy must also include anger and grief work as well as addressing the underlying shame. It is rarely possible to address these issues systematically because they come up as the memory is processed. Flexibility on the part of the therapist and a willingness to reintroduce concepts as they are needed are important.

Increased Integration

In the past, many therapists spent large amounts of time with each alter, processing memories and doing therapy. As more has been learned about the nature of DID, therapists have generally approached individual alters more within the context of the unified Self. DID clients are individual people who experience their minds as consisting of separate personalities that are able to function autonomously. Yet they are single persons. Consequently, any therapy needs to be done with the concept of increased awareness in mind. Interaction with individual alters is essential to successful therapy with a DID client, but the therapist's decisions about what interactions are appropriate will always be based on whether the intervention is likely to lead in the direction of more integrated functioning. Any treatment that is likely to lead to further dissociation is inappropriate.

One example of an intervention that would lead to more integrated functioning is for a therapist to comment when she notices a shift in the client's affect, speech, or physical presentation and to simply ask the client to notice what just happened. Another helpful intervention is for a therapist to look for situations in which he can reinforce that alters are all parts of the same person by saying such things as, "I can see that a part of you is feeling sad." An example of an intervention that is likely to lead to further dissociation is for a therapist to encourage a dissociator to share in depth about past trauma before helping the client to create containment techniques for managing the emotions. Another example is for a therapist to ally himself with a particular alter or keep secrets from others within the system. This behavior reinforces the client's belief that some parts are better than others or that people on the outside cannot be trusted, which only serves to increase internal conflict.

Addressing Anger

Addressing anger is important during the trauma stage of therapy as well. The typical DID client carries her anger in the form of one or more ego states. Sometimes one part unleashes her anger on others (including the therapist), and sometimes she unleashes it on the host by barraging her with insults and other verbal attacks.

> I have three office rules: clients cannot physically hurt themselves, my office, or me. They can talk, draw, yell, sing, and so forth. If the system does not trust any alter to keep that rule, it needs to contain that part internally until it can contract to keep the rules. My office is a safe space. I cannot be a person's therapist if she breaks these safety rules. I repeat this statement, as necessary, until understood by all.
> (Maggie, therapist, Virginia)

Sometimes a client's anger is acted out through self-injury or reckless behaviors. Eating disorders and chemical abuse are common ways for dissociators to both cope with strong emotions and punish the host. Yet if the therapist attempts to talk to the host about her anger, it will often be met with denial. As far as she is concerned, there is no anger. "Maybe Jenny (the rebellious adolescent part) is angry, but that is not me," the host might say. There are several reasons for this reaction. One is that feelings tend to be overwhelming for dissociators. Anger may feel especially threatening because it has probably been seen in perpetrators in the past. It is doubtful that a dissociator wants to act in ways that her abusers did. If anything, she wants to distance herself from their behaviors. Yet abuse survivors often carry *introjects* (mental representations of their abusers) with them. This fact is nothing to be ashamed of. It is a normal outcome of victimization, but it can cause continued victimization for the dissociator if she carries the negative impact and behavior of the abuser with her and, as a result, acts out in inappropriate ways toward herself or others.

If the dissociator recognizes this anger within herself, it must seem frightening at times. Her earliest experiences with anger were likely to have been with people who lost control and raged. She may believe that this behavior is the only option available to her if she begins to acknowledge her own anger. In therapy, however, she will learn new ways of managing emotions in an environment in which safety can be created first. Her anger may essentially feel overwhelming, she may fear being anything like the perpetrator(s), and she has not yet learned how to manage the anger. Consequently, she fears losing control. Finally, allowing specific parts to carry the anger has probably worked on her behalf. It is not unusual for a dissociative woman to have an angry male part who can come forward to protect her. Amazingly enough, some of the angriest protectors are child parts who have learned to act like bullies in an attempt to keep others safe. It can be helpful for both the therapist and the client to realize that the angriest alters are often scared children. These alters have learned to use anger as a way of feeling more powerful and of keeping potential abusers away. That is creative thinking for a child. The therapist's job is to help the client see that although this behavior was ingenious at the time of the abuse, it is really not appropriate for a child alter to feel that she has to be in charge now. Approached that way, how can the system as a whole begin to share the responsibility of dealing with the anger?

In addition is the issue of why the client is angry. It is hard to imagine a survivor of childhood abuse not feeling angry. First, there is the issue of what was done to her. Closely associated is the acknowledgment of what has been lost. For most clients, there is anger at self, intertwined with beliefs such as "I must have done something to cause this abuse." The dissociator has probably directed the anger at herself for most of her life. When wounded in childhood, she did not have the ability to separate herself from the abuse. She had to believe that it was happening because of her: "If only I were better. It is my fault that he's so mad." This self-anger is also a way for the child to survive. If she can blame the abuse on herself and her own bad behavior, it means she also has the power to stop the abuse. She simply needs to change her behavior. This thinking is what Colin Ross refers to as the locus of control shift.[2] Not until later in therapy will she truly be able to shift her thinking to the point where her anger can be directed at the person who hurt her. It is at this point that many life questions begin to surface, as the client begins wrestling with the realization that much suffering exists in this life. Making sense of that suffering, and turning it into personal growth, is a huge task that continues throughout therapy.

INTEGRATION WORK

The next stages of integration and postintegration are closely tied together. *Integration* is a process, as opposed to an actual event, that begins as soon as DID-focused therapy begins. To view integration simply as a time when all the internal parts come together to form a unified self does not do justice to the process. It ignores the tremendous amount of grief work that has taken place before any fusing of parts. This work involves grief that is related to the abuse and the effects it has had on the client's life as well as grief that is related to the abandonment the individual experienced as a child and has continued to carry into adulthood. During the trauma work, as these issues are addressed, there will be an integration of memories that were previously held by specific parts. In addition, there will be empathy and grief that is shared among parts as they begin to heal from their pain. Some of the most poignant work that occurs is when the host begins to realize that other parts have been protecting her by holding her pain. Then, as the client moves into the next stage and continues to integrate memories, she may begin to notice that she is not hearing distinct voices in her head anymore. She might notice that parts are still there, but that they operate more closely together. A kind of blending begins to take place.

> I still notice parts. Maybe it is a facial expression I catch in the mirror. Maybe it is a brief laugh that reminds me of somebody younger from a long time ago. I do not switch anymore, though. If another part is present, I am right there with her. We didn't decide it would be this way. It just happened. I noticed one day that it was quiet inside my head. The silence was so deafening that it startled me. That's what integration is to me.
> (Lisa, client, Minneapolis)

Planned Fusion and Integration

There are many views of integration among both therapists and clients. Ultimately, it is the client who must decide which option to choose. The most commonly accepted approach centers on the belief that individual parts must fuse together to become one. Some therapists use very concrete methods for facilitating this process.

Jill decided she wanted to merge with a younger part. It was a joint decision, and the whole system was in agreement. Her therapist talked a lot about process and things happening as they needed to, but Jill wanted none of that. "We're integrating. That's what we've decided to do," she said. Once they talked it through, the therapist decided that Jill knew what she was doing and that she was taking a step forward in her healing. So, at Jill's request, they planned a little integration ceremony. Toni, the younger part, said her good-byes. The two talked about what they would be gaining by joining together, and Jill read a poem that Toni especially liked. Then the two held hands in Jill's mind. Each chose a color of paint, and as the therapist walked them through the process of joining, Jill and Toni watched their paint colors begin to mix together to create something new. When Jill opened her eyes she reported that she could feel Toni, but that she was very much a part of herself.

In this case, a structured technique was appropriate and helpful. The client made the decision, and it fit her personality and preferences. The biggest caution for therapists taking this approach is to not be so quick to do integration "rituals" that the client feels pushed into premature action. If the client feels pushed, she may do whatever she can to please the therapist. Then, instead of true fusion taking place, alters simply go into hiding. Therapists also want to guard against creating any unnecessary dependence in which the client feels she needs a therapist's direction to facilitate any forward movement. It is also important that therapists do not unconsciously send a message that the goal of the therapy is simply to fuse internal parts. If therapist and client work as partners, it is less likely that will happen. When fusion does occur, if the client finds it helpful to do something symbolic to mark the event, the therapist should allow her to design something that carries personal meaning. Many creative, client-motivated techniques have been used to facilitate the integration process, from blending colors to writing symphonies to creating artwork that represents the internal process taking place.

Spontaneous Fusion and Integration

Another belief about integration is that the final merging of parts occurs spontaneously, which is related to the earlier comment that integration is a process that is occurring throughout therapy. This approach takes the stance that a final goal of integration is not really the issue. Instead, integration of memory leads to increased awareness among parts. As parts continue to grow in awareness and operate more consciously, fusions among parts gradually begin to take place. The overall therapy goal is continued integration of the Self, as with the more structured approach, but much greater responsibility is put on the client in terms of how the process will play itself out.

Co-Consciousness

Another option is for the client to continue to live as a person with DID, but as one who operates co-consciously. In other words, the parts are still separate, but they work together as one functioning system. The difference between this and the pretherapy system is increased awareness. Instead of switching to allow each part to function, the parts communicate, share space, and make decisions together. They operate as a united front, and no one on the outside is the wiser. Some clients choose this option out of respect for their various parts and the tremendous work they have done over the years, believing it is more important to share the space and operate as an internal family. Others feel that the fusion of parts is much like a death, even though these are parts of one Self, so they choose to allow them to remain separate. The questions are whether memory and awareness are becoming more integrated and whether the client is able to lead a more independent and fulfilled life. The overall goal in therapy is to create a more integrated Self, which leads to more integrated functioning. Although there is not just one way of manifesting that experience, this approach often works more effectively as a temporary outcome, because it can easily lead to further dissociation in the face of severe stress.

POSTINTEGRATION THERAPY

When a client is able to operate as a unified Self, either through fusion of parts or internal cooperation, for a distinct period of time, with continuous memory throughout that time, it is generally appropriate to move into *postintegration therapy*. Again, the stages of therapy are fluid and are delineated here to provide a treatment framework for the therapist. The concept of a postintegration stage creates the space for solidifying coping methods that have been learned throughout therapy as alternatives to dissociation. It is also the time for learning the life skills needed to live without dissociation. Although these skills are taught throughout therapy, they will be solidified during the final stage. Working with cognitive distortions is an important part of this stage, and educating the client about "real life" becomes a mainstay of the work that occurs in therapy. Helping clients adopt a realistic view of life is important. Many clients carry the belief that once a final fusion of internal parts takes place, they will be "cured," so to speak. It can be difficult for clients to accept that life as a single, unified Self also brings with it degrees of suffering. Clients may carry a certain naiveté about their abilities to navigate life's stormy seas once integration has occurred. This

1. As you learn to communicate internally, take a roll call before each session and find out what each part needs from the session.
2. Ask for what you need. Do not assume that the therapist can read your mind. If the therapist is moving too quickly and you are feeling overwhelmed, tell her you need to slow down.
3. Recognize that no one person, not even your therapist, can provide all the support for your needs.
4. Ask for feedback if you are not sure why your therapist is doing something or if she says something that feels hurtful or confusing.

Figure 5.2 Client Tips for Becoming an Active Partner in Therapy

stage, however, is also a time of empowerment. L. S. Dickstein defines empowerment as "the process by which a victim's individual decisions lead to personal growth and increased strength."[3] This stage of therapy is a time for rebuilding after having lost so much.

Clients often experience this stage as a time for learning about relationships and about how they, as individuals, fit into the world. They will begin to see themselves as whole persons, complete with strengths and weaknesses and positive and negative impulses, and confronting the same issues as the people around them. When faced with situations that feel overwhelming, they will also find themselves experiencing a full range of emotions without dissociating. They will find that there are many things about themselves that need to be honored as they move out of the victim role and into the role of "member of the human race." Most clients discover that this rather ordinary role brings with it choices and wonderment they did not even know existed before. This time is the time for growing into their adult selves as they begin to truly incorporate their own beliefs and values into their daily lives. This time is the moment when the butterfly emerges from the cocoon in all its splendor. (See Figure 5.2.)

Chapter Six

When Seeing a Therapist Is Not Enough

Heather has been in therapy for four years and is feeling "stuck." She is tired of talking about her childhood abuse, yet she feels unable to manage day-to-day life without the safety net of her weekly sessions. Heather's therapist feels that the focus needs to be on the "here and now" so that she can learn how to better manage the emotions that create so much difficulty in her life. Heather agrees with that goal, yet week after week, nothing seems to change.

Many DID patients find that they reach a sort of impasse in therapy that requires additional intervention. For some, this point presents itself early in therapy in the form of flashbacks and suicidal thoughts that become so intrusive that hospitalization or some other form of physical intervention is required. For others such as Heather, it is simply a matter of feeling "stuck."

THERAPIST FIT

Clients feel stuck in therapy for many reasons. Sometimes the therapist is simply not an appropriate fit. That does not have to mean that he is unskilled in his work. Perhaps the client and therapist are personality mismatches, which may leave the DID client feeling unsafe with sharing certain issues in sessions. Or perhaps the therapist's style is not quite what the client seeks. Even when therapists are operating from the same theoretical background and using similar techniques, each will have his own personal style. Thus, a client may find it helpful to decide prior to therapy what type of person she wants. That still might not guarantee an ideal fit, but it will help the client to feel that she has more control in the process. Let's suppose a client has been in therapy for a while, like Heather. She has been relatively happy with both the therapist and the process, yet she finds herself feeling stuck nonetheless. What might that mean?

Feeling stuck is quite subjective. To one person, it might mean going to sessions week after week and processing no new information. For another person, it might mean another bout with panic attacks and not understanding why old behaviors have returned. For some, it is the frustration of still being in therapy after five years while believing that everything should be "normal" by now. The list is probably as long as the number of people who are currently in treatment for DID. Understanding some of the reasons for getting stuck, however, will help both client and therapist avoid the situation or at least manage it more effectively when it occurs.

Getting stuck in therapy is not much different from driving in the winter. You can be cruising along and feeling confident, then you hit a patch of ice and wake up to find yourself sitting in a ditch. If you have planned for the possibility of getting stuck, however, your survival kit will be close at hand and movement will soon be possible again.

What pushes someone off course in therapy? First of all, getting stuck may simply be a normal part of the therapy process. It helps clients to incorporate new coping skills and healthier ways of thinking. Irvin Yalom, an existential psychiatrist, teaches that a genuine relationship between therapist and client is the most important ingredient in healing.[1] Getting stuck is a great way for clients to learn how to be more genuine with another human being because they are forced to learn to talk about things that may be creating conflict between themselves and their therapists and they can begin to learn how to ask for help in an appropriate way. In other words, therapy is a process, and getting stuck may just be a part of the process. Yet there is no virtue in being unnecessarily stuck; there must be reasons that someone might find herself feeling stuck in her own therapeutic process.

INTERNAL CONFLICTS

Movement in therapy is sometimes stalled because of internal conflicts. Internal parts may have different goals. While one part is trying to process memories and move toward integration, another may be purposely sabotaging the treatment in some way. A therapist may find herself entangled in power struggles with an alter only to realize later that she has been steered completely off course.

Internal parts sometimes guard their territories aggressively. These parts are formed to play a role, and that role is generally associated with carrying specific memories or feelings. If a client is talking about work relationships and a desire to be more assertive, the goal might seem very clear unless, of course, there is an ego state that carries the feeling of anger so that the host does not have to do so. In sessions, the client may talk about various work situations and possibilities for acting more assertively in those situations. Both the client and therapist are feeling positive about the sessions and the way things have been progressing in therapy. One day, however, the client comes in talking about her internal voices. Another situation had occurred at work in which she had felt taken advantage of. She could hear the swearing and screaming inside. She says, "I cannot assert myself in situations like that. I'll lose control." "And what does 'lose control' mean?" the therapist asks. "I might say something terrible and get fired," she responds. As the two explore the situation together, it becomes apparent that there is a part of the client that is angry and does not trust herself to deal with the situation. After all, she has always been passive in the past. The therapist helps her to talk things through, and after some internal communication, the angry part admits she feels misunderstood by others: "I'm not a mean person, but somebody has to protect her (the host). Besides, I don't want to die. If she starts taking care of everything she won't need me anymore."

This moment is the time for some education and reassurance. First, the goal of therapy has nothing to do with getting rid of parts. It is about operating in a more integrated fashion. Second, internal parts, however many, are all aspects of one self, and although they may feel very separate, there is still only one body. So, how can they work together? Every part plays an important role in creating the whole. When two parts appear to be diametrically opposed, the therapist can remind the client of this example of ambivalence. What person hasn't experienced ambivalence in her life? The goal at this point is to learn to manage these feelings; then the client can return to the work-related issues and continue to move forward.

Internal conflicts, or resistance, are a primary reason conflicts between therapists and their dissociative clients, as well as a feeling on the part of the client that she is unable to continue in a certain direction, arise. Some therapists consider client resistance to be extremely negative, and when therapy is not going well, the excuse is always about client resistance. That position can be both unfortunate and disrespectful to the client. When the term *resistance* is used, it is in a neutral, nonjudgmental stance. When conflicting ego states interfere with the stated therapy goals or when they sabotage a session, it is helpful to view that behavior as a clear signal that the alters want to be heard. If it is assumed that each part wants the best for the system as a whole, it becomes much easier to hear what is trying to be communicated. When those thoughts and feelings are addressed, the system is able to function much more effectively.

Another issue that commonly occurs internally is in the area of memory. In childhood, individual parts did a superb job of protecting the body. The way the host has been able to survive and function in the adult world is by keeping those memories dissociated from her consciousness. It is only logical to assume that there would be fear associated with memories being shared among parts. It is very common for internal parts to take the Jack Nicholson "You can't handle the truth" approach with the host, similar to his rigid military stance portrayed in the film *A Few Good Men*. Consequently, conflict is to be expected during the trauma work. The conflicts are meant to protect.

DEFENSES

Defense mechanisms may also contribute to why a client is feeling stuck. Defense mechanisms are unconcious psychological processes used to keep anxiety away from the conscious mind. They are also protective behaviors. If a client intellectualizes to avoid dealing with emotions she perceives to be overwhelming, the defense operates as a kind of psychic barrier. We all use defense mechanisms, and we tend to gravitate toward the same ones across time. Because these behaviors are unconscious, though, we are generally unaware of when we are employing them. Defenses, then, become a therapy issue. As the therapist observes defenses at work, he is able to begin, slowly, to help the client become more aware of how she uses these defenses to protect herself. The purpose is not to pull away her protection, but to help her understand herself more clearly and to learn more adaptive ways of coping. As a client develops more ego strength (the ability to regulate feelings and actions even when experiencing extreme stress), there is less need to rely on these defenses, including dissociation.

CONFLICTS WITH THE THERAPIST

Conflicts with the therapist might also cause a client to feel as if her therapy progress is being stalled. Conflicts might be very clear-cut. There might be a personality conflict or disagreement on an issue that needs to be resolved, so until the issue is addressed, the client feels stuck. Typically, however, the issue is much deeper than that. Many therapy conflicts are related to the transference relationship (when a client transfers aspects of prior relationships, especially parental, onto the therapist). Such transference is actually positive in that the confines of a therapy session can provide the emotional safety needed to begin to explore the relational issues that have affected the dissociator throughout her life. What can feel like no movement may, in reality, be the exact movement she needs for personal growth at the time. Most people go though life without addressing the unconscious influences on their behaviors until they are in situations in which the pain is either severe enough or disabling enough that confronting these issues becomes necessary. The pain, then, eventually becomes the healer. It is like the person in recovery who introduces himself by saying, "I am a grateful alcoholic." He is not grateful that he almost drank himself to death or, for that matter, that he can never drink again. He is grateful that the pain of alcoholism provided him with the vehicle for obtaining the kind of life he did not even know existed before. The pain became the healer.

Pain, as healer, is pain nonetheless, however, and often the issues that need to be discussed are difficult at best. Some issues create so much anxiety that clients will do whatever they can to avoid the topic. It is not unusual for a therapist to start down a certain path with a client and have that person skillfully turn him in a different direction. Sometimes internal parts come forward to divert attention away from the troubling topic. Sometimes the client dissociates, becomes argumentative, or starts talking about superfluous things. As the therapist gets to know a client better, he becomes more attuned to the distractions, or roadblocks, the client is most likely to use along the way. It can be frustrating at times to both the client and the therapist when these things happen. Typically, what is occurring for the client is ambivalence. For example, she may want to talk about a rape that occurred when she was fourteen years old, but the anxiety associated with the incident is itself frightening. There may be a fear of overwhelming emotion or shame about the incident; furthermore, there may be a desire to keep herself safe, which is good. Yet she knows there will have to be some pain if she expects to work through the issue. If the therapist can frame the resistance in a positive way and consider the ambivalence he might be feeling in a similar situation, it will help the client to deal with her own frustration in this situation so that the lack of movement does not turn into a power struggle.

Therapist frustration is a reality. Therapists can create problems for themselves if they pretend that all their feelings in the therapeutic relationship are positive. Therapists are human and thus have human feelings and responses to what they are experiencing. When situations occur in therapy that cause movement to be thwarted, many things can happen. The ideal situation, of course, is that the therapist will see exactly what is taking place to cause the client's resistance and will intervene in such a way that the client will see what is happening and move past it, and whatever issue is at hand will be resolved. The more experienced the therapist is at treating DID and the longer the relationship has been, the more likely that will happen. Yet because we live in an imperfect world, at times a therapist in this situation will think the client is manipulating her and thus might feel angry. Or she may feel frustrated that every time a particular subject comes up, the discussion gets sidetracked. The therapist may even begin to question her own therapeutic skills. It is important for therapists to be able to honestly look at these issues and how they might be impacting therapy. Doing so can be a great help in bringing the client back to the original goal.

FEAR

Somewhat related to the fear of a particular issue is the fear of moving forward. Clients may fear that getting better means they will have to end therapy and lose the therapeutic relationship. Like all relationships, the therapeutic relationship will end someday, but barring some unforeseen circumstance, it will not end before the client is ready. This fear may have to do with attachment issues that originated in childhood. The individual with DID has not always been able to rely on others. Many dissociators have experienced neglect or trauma at an early age at the hands of others, quite possibly caregivers that they should have been able to trust. That abandonment experience in childhood may have felt like a death, and those feelings are then revisited with the therapist. This experience can be used as a means of exploring the client's feelings associated with the childhood trauma. The therapist can begin to talk to the client about the importance of living in the present moment. Because we do not know what the future holds, we do not have control over it, but we can make choices for ourselves along the way. One of those choices is when to quit therapy. If integration occurs, therapy does not necessarily end. In fact, postintegration work is necessary for completing the process. When someone has lived her entire life using dissociation as a defense, new skills have to be learned to live life successfully in a more integrated or cooperative state. The decision of when to end therapy will resolve itself, as do most situations in life, if we just do our part by showing up and living in an engaged fashion.

STRESS

Another issue that stops movement is fatigue, although it is often difficult for clients to accept. DID therapy is hard work, and clients sometimes need a break from the in-depth part of that work. At those

Table 6.1 Symptoms of Toxic Stress

Physical	Psychological	Social
Headaches	Anxiety	Relationship problems
Stomach upset	Irritability	Work difficulties
Muscle tension	Agitation	Isolation
Sleep problems	Difficulty concentrating	
Changes in appetite		

times, the therapist might work with the client on self-nurturing skills. Dissociators generally have to learn how to recognize when the stress in their lives has become too great. Thus, at those times, the therapist can talk about the physical and emotional signs of toxic stress and teach basic stress management skills. This work is not stalled therapy. It is an important learning situation that will benefit the client for the rest of her life.

Stress is the body's response to any demand made on it. A certain amount of stress is normal and needed, but if it lasts too long or becomes too severe, the situation becomes toxic. Table 6.1 lists some common symptoms of toxic stress. It is important to be aware of how stress manifests itself in your own life.

TRANSITIONS

Finally, it is helpful to recognize that therapy, like life, consists of transitional periods. A client may find herself spending weeks, or even months, working on a particular issue to the point of resolution and then hitting a plateau where it feels as if she is no longer making progress. The plateau, though, offers her a chance to process the previous experience and regroup, so to speak. This time is also when she may actually grieve the loss of old behaviors or the letting go of an issue that she has carried with her for many years. Yes, there is loss in giving up old behaviors, even if those behaviors were unhealthy. There is also a reidentification of self that occurs throughout the therapy process. Initially, the dissociator may question who she is as she struggles with the initial diagnosis of DID. Then she continues to ask that question as she processes memories and gives up old coping behaviors in favor of new, more adaptive ways of being. The transitional periods offer her an opportunity to reevaluate who she is, grieve her losses, and stop and rest without having to abandon the therapeutic safety net along the way.

INTERVENTIONS

Often, the issues discussed above resolve themselves as they are addressed, but occasionally they do not. At these times, an intervention of some sort may help create movement. Getting stuck has nothing to do with failure, nor is it about blame. The therapist and client are working together and when one person in the relationship feels stuck, it affects both. In addition, at times the therapist can feel just as stuck as the client does. Thus, consider using the situation as an opportunity for individual growth and a strengthening of the therapeutic relationship.

Consultation

One way of addressing getting stuck is through consultation with another mental health professional. In this situation, someone with expertise in the treatment of DID is chosen to hear what both the therapist and client perceive the problem to be. The consulting therapist can help both see possibilities that may have been overlooked because the therapist and client are so close to the issues at hand. Sometimes this third person ends up becoming a backup therapist for the client as well, creating a safety net for the client so that she has consistency with her therapy when her own therapist is out of town or is otherwise unavailable. It may also offer her the opportunity to access specific treatments that her own therapist does not use, such as eye movement desensitization and reprocessing (EMDR) or art therapy. If the client and the therapists are willing to work together, with clear boundaries, an excellent opportunity for continued growth can be provided.

Another way to become unstuck is through the use of adjunctive therapies. There are many adjunctive therapies and techniques, but some of the most common include DBT, hypnosis, art therapy, EMDR, bodywork, group therapy, and meditation, which are all discussed later in this chapter.

TRAUMA SYMPTOMS

Feeling stuck is just one reason clients may find themselves needing more than a weekly therapy session. A dissociator knows that some of the most troubling aspects of therapy are about having to deal with the trauma symptoms that occur. Most notable are the flashbacks, panic attacks, and continued dissociation that occurs for clients when they feel threatened.

Flashbacks

It has been said that dissociation is not as much about the past as it is about a fear of living in the present. That is true, but the effects of the past are carried into the present. One's physical being is affected by severe prolonged trauma, and the body does not automatically return to normal functioning just because the trauma has ended. Flashbacks are an example.

> Sue has learned that she cannot watch movies where she'll witness sexual violence. If she is in a theater and a violent scene comes on, she goes out to the lobby and does some deep breathing for a few minutes before returning to the movie. She knows that if she does not do that, she risks the possibility of having a flashback of a time when she was brutally raped as a teen. She knows because it has happened many times before. The response itself is physiological. The brain takes in the image on the screen, searches its memory files, and realizes that something similar has happened to this body. Sue begins to experience the same sense of panic as in the past, and her body goes into a fight or flight response as she notices the familiar queasiness rising in her stomach. She starts blinking rapidly as images of her own rape flash through her mind, pictures so vivid it is like turning the pages of a photo album. Before therapy, the images were so invasive that Sue would become nonfunctional for days at a time. Since therapy, she has learned to slow herself down with breathing techniques that she practices several times a week. Then she reminds herself, "That was then and this is now. I am not in any danger."
>
> Courtney, on the other hand, has not been as successful at managing her flashbacks. She becomes so overwhelmed by the feelings associated with the images that she begins to dissociate before allowing herself the opportunity to practice her coping skills. Typically, the flashbacks start, she feels overwhelmed, she dissociates to manage the feelings, and then an-

other part comes forward to take over. Because Courtney's dissociation is so automatic, she does not stick around long enough when feeling threatened to see if there really is any danger. Unfortunately, if this dissociation happens often, due to some kind of external stressor, the emotional and physiological stress of the flashbacks takes its toll on her body and ability to function. At that point, in-depth therapy is not possible. Coping becomes the primary issue.

Anxiety

Panic attacks are another reaction to the present having its roots in the past, for two reasons. One is physiological. As discussed in chapter 1, prolonged trauma causes physiological changes in the body. Then, even years after experiencing the trauma, the body may still react to perceived threats as if the original trauma is occurring. The response ends up becoming an overreaction, because the body's internal fight or flight mechanism has been activated. The other reason panic occurs is because the dissociator may fear much of what she encounters in life in the present. The perceived threat is the issue, however.

Let's assume we are sitting in my living room having a cup of tea when my new little puppy runs into the room. Being a puppy, we see his puppy nature in full bloom. He chases his ball. He jumps. He barks. I pat my hands on my lap and call to him, "Come on, puppy, jump!" As I turn toward you, however, assuming you are sharing in this revelry, I see a look of fear instead. I am surprised. After all, this dog is a tiny puppy, not an adult pit bull. When I ask you about the fear, you tell me about the time you were six years old and a dog attacked you as you were riding your bike home from school. Then I begin to understand your reaction. Your brain is registering danger based on a past experience, and you go with the perceived threat instead of slowing yourself down long enough to assess the situation.

For some people anxiety, to some degree, becomes the first response to situations in life because life seems so threatening. Past memories become so encompassing that everything feels dangerous. Even if that is a dissociator's experience, it can change. Life can be enjoyed. Clients can learn to let down their guards and begin to breathe freely for possibly the first time in their lives.

Dissociation

Continued dissociation is another coping defense that can hinder movement. Dissociation occurs at different levels, with DID being the most extreme form of dissociation, but dissociation itself is not unusual. We all do it to some degree. The hindrance occurs when it becomes automatic, a first line of defense. The reasons are obvious. If someone shuts down the minute he feels threatened, he will miss opportunities for learning how to manage his emotions and responses to life. If the dissociation occurs on a regular basis in therapy, it prevents the client from addressing important issues. A therapist can work with a client on ways to manage the dissociation and can also help the dissociator to develop new coping skills, but she cannot take away the client's dissociative defenses, nor should she try. The client and therapist need to work together to explore why the client is reluctant to stay present in a session when feeling threatened. Is it fear of the topic? Is dissociation a way of feeling more control? Does it happen because she gives her power to the therapist, resulting in playing a passive role in which she begins to feel victimized? Or has it merely become a habit that needs to be replaced with other behaviors? Bear in mind that dissociation will be the first line of defense early in therapy because it is all that the client knows, but sometimes there is a reliance on dissociation as a defense after other skills have been learned. At that point, the dissociator has to ask herself what is being gained by hanging on to this defense and, conversely, what will be lost if she gives up the defense. There are very real grief issues associated with making behavioral changes. The client needs to allow herself to acknowledge how difficult it can be to accept life on life's terms. Then she will be in a place where she can allow herself to experience how joyous it can be to do the same.

ADJUNCTIVE THERAPIES

Weekly sessions with a therapist may be good, helpful, and effective, but when a client is feeling stuck, she may need more. The additional help is called adjunctive therapy. Some of the most commonly used adjunctive therapies helpful in terms of treating DID are art therapy, DBT, meditation, EMDR, group therapy, bodywork, and hypnosis. Some of these techniques a therapist can incorporate into regular therapy sessions. Others are therapies that the client will be referred to in addition to the regular therapy sessions. In the next section, I will briefly describe each of these interventions and why they might be used.

Art Therapy

Some therapists use art therapy as a part of their sessions. For some people, art is a way of communicating things they do not feel able to communicate verbally. In the case of DID, if some parts are non-verbal, they may be willing to draw memories or other information they want the system or the therapist to know.

A therapist might refer a client to an art therapy group as a way of accessing information or parts that are reluctant to come forward. A therapist might even give a client an art assignment to help internal parts to work together and begin to share thoughts and feelings they hold individually. A therapist might give assignments to systems as a whole to work on collages about a specific issue or time in the client's life. Clients can do daily art journals in contrast to the usual written journals they might be doing. If a client is stuck, a therapist can even ask her to illustrate the issue at hand; the therapist simply switches gears in the middle of the session, hands the client some paper, lets her choose whether to use colored pencils, crayons, or some other medium, and then gives the assignment. Afterward, the client titles the work, and the discussion goes on from there.

Art therapy is a specialized field. Therapists need to seek out people who are trained in this area and obtain appropriate supervision if they want to make the most of the use of art in their sessions. It is inappropriate to use art therapy as a diagnostic tool without proper training. Many clients open up with this work because it accesses a part of the self that is rarely acknowledged, not to mention that it is fun.

Dialectical Behavioral Therapy

Marsha Linehan developed dialectical behavior therapy, or DBT, as a structured treatment for borderline personality disorder (BPD).[2] Its basic tenets include the following:

1. The interrelatedness of individual behavior patterns. In other words, a person's behavior affects both self and others, and the opposite is true as well.
2. The fundamental nature of reality is change and process. Nothing is static; things are always changing.

3. The importance of developing "wise mind." Emotional experience plus logical analysis plus intuitive knowing equals wise mind.
4. The development of mindfulness skills for achieving wise mind. To be mindful is to be aware of the present moment and to accept it without judgment.

One of the features of DID is emotional dysregulation. One of the goals of DBT is to teach clients the skills they need for managing emotions. The structure of the therapy is also good because it helps clients to stay on task, rather than getting sidetracked by their own emotions or the drama of life. DBT workshops are available to therapists on a regular basis, as are DBT supervision groups. Linehan's book, *Cognitive-Behavioral Treatment of Borderline Personality Disorder*, and her related workbook, *Skills Training Manual for Treating Borderline Personality Disorder*, are available at most major bookstores as well. The information in the workbook is very helpful and can be used regularly with clients during sessions. A therapist may, however, suggest a DBT group as opposed to working on the principles in individual sessions. A group provides the opportunity for clients to learn new skills that can be used for a lifetime. The emotional regulation skills will also help clients experience more success in their individual sessions. Having another therapist involved in the treatment is also an added plus. No one person can be all that we want or need. Individuals can gain valuable insights about themselves by including more people in the treatment.

Clients should not allow themselves to be deterred by the BPD label. These skills are valuable for anyone. Addressing the behaviors and other issues that are affecting the dissociator in the here and now is much more important than focusing on a diagnosis. The therapist will deal with diagnostic issues and, it is hoped, discuss her impressions with her client, but the nuts and bolts of therapy are about changing troublesome beliefs and behaviors so that the client can live a happier and more productive life. DBT training can provide the basic tools for doing just that.

Mindfulness Meditation

A technique very complementary to DBT is mindfulness meditation. This concept is somewhat new to therapy, but it is gaining in popularity because of its usefulness in managing emotions. Jon Kabat-Zinn developed a mindfulness-based meditation program at the University of Massachusetts Medical Center for use with patients suffering from terminal illnesses and chronic pain.[3] Both DBT and mindfulness meditation teach the importance of staying in the present moment and the acceptance of yourself without judgment. A therapist might even want to learn mindfulness meditation and begin practicing it in her own life before deciding when and how to use the practice with clients. Besides acceptance and living in the here and now, mindfulness techniques can help clients connect more with their bodies through the use of techniques such as yoga and body scan.

Of course, therapists need to use wisdom in terms of when mindfulness meditation might be appropriate for a client. If a client is extremely fragmented and in the beginning stages of therapy, extensive meditation can be harmful and can even create further fragmentation. If the meditation is practiced in a religious setting, it might even remind some clients of past abuse, which could lead to retraumatization. Instead, a therapist might introduce only the basic concepts of mindfulness—staying in the present, accepting what is happening without judgment, and focusing on the breath—until the client reaches a stage of therapy in which she is more integrated.

Therapists also need to be mindful of their client's belief systems, preferences, and states of consciousness. Some clients react adversely to the Buddhist teaching that has influenced the development of DBT and most mindfulness-based programs, whereas others embrace the teaching and find it helpful. It is inappropriate for a therapist to promote her own spiritual beliefs in therapy or to be disrespectful of a client's beliefs; this should be obvious but to some people it is not. When a concept such as mindfulness is introduced to a client, it must be done so with a clear therapeutic goal in mind, such as reducing anxiety. It must also be used within the client's framework, be it secular or spiritual in nature. It would be optimal for a DID client to be able to practice mindfulness skills in a group setting with a therapist specifically trained in this area. The Jon Kabat-Zinn model is especially helpful because it has been adapted to fit the medical community.

Eye Movement Desensitization and Reprocessing

Developed by Francine Shapiro,[4] eye movement desensitization and reprocessing (EMDR) is used to process information, including traumatic material, more quickly than with traditional therapy. Therapists must be specifically trained regarding the use of EMDR with dissociation. In an EMDR session, a client will be asked to think about a bothersome memory, and the therapist will then use one of various techniques to create bilateral stimulation of the brain. These techniques include such things as waving the fingers in front of the client's eyes, tapping the client's hands, having the client hold vibrating sensory pads, or having a client wear a headset while listening to alternating tones. Any of these techniques are acceptable and will produce the same results. The goal is to reduce the intensity of the memory and to change the negative belief associated with the memory into a positive one. Many therapists incorporate EMDR into sessions as needed. If a therapist is not trained in

EMDR but thinks it might be helpful, it is perfectly fine for a client to see a primary therapist and an EMDR therapist at the same time. The client should sign a release form so the therapists can converse about how best to coordinate the treatment. Therapists treating dissociative clients must have advanced training in EMDR and a solid understanding of the dissociative process. It could be harmful for some clients to do EMDR if it is performed too early in the treatment process or by someone unfamiliar with treating dissociation.

Group Therapy

A therapist might suggest a therapy group in addition to individual sessions. There is disagreement among mental health professionals as to whether group therapy is effective for clients with DID. Those who favor it say it can be helpful to have the additional therapy and it is good to be able to share your story with other people who truly understand what it is like to live with DID. Those who are more cautious say that hearing others' stories might be retraumatizing for some individuals. Some suggest that a few clients with borderline features might get into competition with each other for who has the most sensational story. What is most important is the client, however: where she is in therapy and how the group is run. Group therapy is discussed in more detail in chapter 8.

A DID group, however, is not the only option. If the client is at a stage in therapy where a group can be beneficial (co-conscious and able to manage triggers), she might go to a group that deals with specific issues she is dealing with in therapy. Besides dialectical behavior training, a therapist might also consider sending a client to a group for depression or anxiety management. Of course, there are support groups for all kinds of difficulties, but managing emotions and dealing with depression and anxiety are pervasive issues among those diagnosed with DID. Discussing these issues openly and honestly with a therapist will help the client to determine whether group therapy is appropriate.

Bodywork

Entire books have been devoted to the various kinds of bodywork. The method chosen may not be nearly as important as the client's comfort with the practitioner. Bodywork includes such things as the following:

1. *Hakomi:* A body-based psychotherapy used to help clients change negative core beliefs.
2. *Neuromuscular therapy:* Using pressure on a client's muscles to break the stress-tension-pain cycle.
3. *Shiatsu:* A technique in which a therapist works on a client's pressure points and on opening the body's energy meridians.
4. *Swedish massage:* A technique used to relax muscles and increase a client's connectedness to the body, while decreasing emotional and physical stress.
5. *Trager:* The use of light, nonintrusive movements that help decrease chronic tension and induce a deep state of relaxation.

I think a therapist must be very careful with different techniques because it is easy to bypass a patients own responsibility and that should never happen. We can only "take over" when absolutely no other options are available. Bodywork, I find, should be used only in later stages of therapy because, to profit from it, a patient must be able to experience feelings and be able to set boundaries. If this technique is used too early it can retraumatize, which is not a treatment goal.
(Therapist, The Netherlands)

The importance of bodywork for someone with DID is that it helps clients reconnect with their bodies and provides them with one avenue in which they can begin to grieve the past. It is not at all unusual for people who are experiencing extreme emotional pain to divert their emotions into the body unconsciously rather than expressing their feelings more directly. When much of that emotional pain is directly related to actual physical or sexual abuse of the body, a person will often dissociate to escape the pain, but the disconnection between conscious mind and body may continue even after the abuse ends. If a person has been physically or sexually abused, she may actually be afraid to connect with her body because of its reminders of the abuse.

> Christa is terrified of sex. She had been sexually abused as a child. Now that she is married, she wants very much to have a sexual relationship with her husband. She thinks about romantic interludes and sometimes even plans intimate dinners together, but invariably, as the emotional intimacy turns into something physical, Christa's body and mind begin to react in ways she feels unable to control. It might be the way he touches her or a certain inflection in his voice, but when something triggers Christa, her body stiffens and she feels as if she wants to cry. Instead, she forces herself to go away inside to someplace safe while her body goes through the motions of the sexual encounter in which she feels obligated to participate. In therapy, Christa talks about how guilty she feels. "I love my husband and I know he would never hurt me. What's wrong with me?"

For people like Christa, the body represents pain and a feeling of being out of control. As children, we do not have control, so dissociating from the body is an ingenious way of learning how to cope. In adulthood, however, that coping mechanism starts to create problems. The goal becomes learning how to reconnect with the body rather than continuing to see it as the enemy. Bodywork, or massage, is one way of doing that. Ideally, someone who dissociates will want to find a bodyworker who has an understanding of trauma. Even better is if the bodyworker understands dissociation as well. It is also important that clients talk with their therapists about any bodywork they plan to do. In the early stages of therapy, bodywork may be too overwhelming for a client and could even be retraumatizing. A therapist can help her client decide when bodywork would be most appropriate and can also help the client create safety for herself emotionally. This help can be useful because if a dissociator allows a complete stranger to touch her body, it may feel unnerving at first; younger parts might feel especially vulnerable and may even feel that they are about to be retraumatized. Thus, internal communication and safety plans are important. It is up to the client to decide how much she will tell the bodyworker about her diagnosis, but she needs to tell enough to know she will be safe. The client also needs to be able to tell the bodyworker what she is experiencing in her own body so that the bodyworker can be aware of what kinds of touch elicit certain types of responses. A client might say, "I need for you to know that I was sexually abused when I was a child. So, sometimes I feel scared when people touch me and I might even dissociate, or space out. If that happens, I might not seem like my usual self. If I need you to stop for a minute, I'll try to say so, but if I seem scared, could you ask if I am okay? If I say no, we just need to stop for a minute so that I can drink some water and take some deep breaths to get grounded. Is that okay with you?"

A client also has the right to ask a bodyworker to not touch her in a certain area of her body if she is feeling uncomfortable that day. She also has the right to keep on as much clothing as she needs to feel safe. The only way a person can truly feel comfortable with bodywork is by doing some research to ensure that she is making a good choice about a bodyworker. Getting a therapist referral is probably the best way of doing so, but interviewing potential bodyworkers is also an appropriate way to gauge comfort level.

In addition, an individual never completely forgets what has happened to her in the past. Sometimes, though, those memories have been dissociated and stored very far away, like stacks of boxes packed away in the corner of a basement. The conscious mind may be surprised by memories that begin to surface during bodywork. Sometimes they will surface as emotions. It is perfectly normal to laugh or cry during bodywork without even knowing why. Or, someone might get an image in her mind that she has not thought of for a long time, if ever. She might even have somatic reactions, a kind of physical flashback, in which the body reacts as though it is currently experiencing past trauma. All these reactions may help a client see that she is processing the aftereffects of past trauma. If something occurs that cannot be explained, such as having the urge to vomit even though nothing bad is happening or the surfacing of a new memory, it is important to try to accept it rather than dissociating and running away mentally or emotionally. Talking about it or focusing on breathing is a way of staying connected to the present until the experience can be processed with the primary therapist.

Hypnosis

Many DID therapists use hypnosis with their clients as a way of soothing or doing memory work in a safe way. Some therapists use hypnosis to elicit memories or bring alters out so that they can make a diagnosis. In the case of a medical emergency, it might be useful to use hypnosis for that purpose, but people usually remember things as they need to do so. When a client has developed a trusting relationship with a therapist, she will begin to show more and more of herself. That is most appropriate because it leaves control with the client. If a therapist is experienced in both hypnosis and the treatment of DID, however, it can be helpful to use hypnosis as a way of teaching clients to self-soothe. It is also a good technique to use when doing memory work because it will help the client contain emotion in a safe way. In addition, as mentioned in chapter 4, hypnosis is an important component of ego-state therapy.

SUMMARY

In this chapter, the various reasons that a client might feel "stuck" in therapy were discussed. These reasons include not having an appropriate fit with a therapist, not seeing enough forward movement, having old behaviors return, reaching a therapeutic plateau, internal conflicts, defense mechanisms and transference issues, conflicts with the therapist, the fear of moving forward, fatigue, and reaching a transition point. The reality that feeling stuck might mean that a client needs to make a change was also pursued. It might also be, however, that the stuck point is actually a necessary place that allows the client to work on some difficult issues or begin to transition to a new area in therapy. Several adjunctive therapies can help clients work through the various roadblocks they may encounter along the way. Not all these techniques will be of interest or even appropriate for all clients in the course of their therapy, but if someone is drawn to a particular therapy, she can discuss it with her primary therapist, decide her reasons for pursuing it, and begin to formulate some initial goals.

Remember that feeling stuck in therapy is only negative if it is allowed to be. Often, the times when we feel the most stuck are also the times when we receive the greatest insights, if we are just willing to wait long enough for the message to become clear. If you are someone who experiences dissociation, it is important for you to take charge of your therapy.

Chapter Seven

How Medication Might Help

Kim had suffered from depression most of her life. It lasted from a couple of weeks to a couple of months and sometimes even longer. Then, as if by magic, her mood would return to normal. The therapist listened as Kim continued her story. "I'm here because I am depressed again and I just can't take it anymore. I've had two years of feeling great and then, for no apparent reason, I wake up one morning feeling so sad that I can't even pull myself out of bed."

The therapist agreed to work with Kim on her depression, but as therapy progressed and Kim revealed more and more of herself, the therapist began to realize that dissociation was also a part of Kim's experience. Six months later, she met an alter, named Kimberly, and diagnosed Kim with dissociative identity disorder.

The therapist, though untrained in the treatment of DID, was eager to jump into trauma work. Her theory was simple: reprocess the trauma, integrate Kim's internal parts, no more depression! As therapy continued, however, the exact opposite occurred. Kim became so depressed that she was unable to continue full-time employment and her suicidal thoughts turned into suicidal gestures. What should the therapist have done?

Wouldn't it be nice to be able to take a pill that would make all your problems go away? Of course, life does not work like that. Even with strictly physical illnesses, healing involves a lot more than popping a pill. It involves patient attitude, the doctor/patient relationship, and often major lifestyle changes. It takes a lot of work to maintain a state of health, and much of that has to do with our intentions. It is no different with DID. A client's first priority is to decide what she really wants as an end result of therapy so that she can focus on that goal. That means making choices that will move her in that direction. It is fine for the goal to change over time; in fact, it probably will.

The usual treatment for DID is psychodynamic therapy, but even the best talk therapy can be more successful if the person seeking treatment is treated as a whole person as opposed to someone who has simply been diagnosed with a disorder. In other words, what does the client need to reach his intended goals? The answer is the use of whatever adjunctive therapies are necessary to address the issues associated with the diagnosis and to consider physical, spiritual, and social needs in addition to the emotional. At this point, medication can become an important addition to the treatment. Medication itself will not cure someone of DID, but it can help her manage the coexisting disorders, such as depression or anxiety, she might be experiencing. It would be highly unusual for someone with DID not to have a mood disorder or multiple physical complaints as well.

Thus, a therapist might refer someone to a psychiatrist for medication for many reasons. One may be to manage the symptoms associated with anxiety or depression. Not only is that important because it offers the person some relief, it also allows her to focus on therapy more easily. Another reason someone might be referred for a medication evaluation is to deal with the intrusive thoughts, suicidal behaviors, flashbacks, or sleep disorders that often accompany posttraumatic stress. Again, medication might offer some relief.

There is no virtue in people suffering miserably if they do not have to do so. If a person has DID, she might not be fully aware at times of how stress is affecting her. A dissociator might also think she does not deserve to feel better. In addition, a certain percentage of dissociators may even believe they were drugged and then abused in the past; consequently, they want nothing to do with medication. If any of these scenarios apply to a client, they need to be addressed with the therapist so that the client can begin to take care of herself appropriately in the present.

When clients meet with a psychiatrist, it is important for them to be as honest as possible. It is helpful to talk with the primary therapist first about the purpose of the psychiatric evaluation and what information needs to be shared with the doctor. It is also helpful to write down what needs to be discussed and then, as questions arise, they can be added to the list. Meeting a new doctor can be stressful, but writing things down will help the client stay focused and grounded.

Some psychiatrists also do therapy, but most do not, and it should not be automatically expected when referred for a medication evaluation. Also, psychiatrists are trained to diagnose, so the doctor will spend time asking questions and using that information to determine the best medications, if any, to prescribe. By the same token, some psychiatrists take a holistic approach and may spend more time with the patient so that they can gain a better understanding of her as a whole person rather than as someone who is merely presenting with a diagnosis such as depression. These doctors may consider using herbal remedies and nutritional interventions as a part of the treatment. If this type of treatment is important to a client, she should actively seek it out.

Typically, a client will return to the psychiatrist every few weeks for checks to assess the effectiveness of the medication and to determine whether any changes need to be made in terms of dosage or the type of medication being taken. Between medication checks, a client will continue to see her individual therapist.

It is also important for a client to see a psychiatrist who understands DID and for the primary therapist to communicate with that psychiatrist as needed; some issues associated with DID are not present with other psychiatric disorders. First, different parts may present with different symptoms, which can create confusion diagnostically. Therefore, the doctor will want to create a picture of who the client is as a whole and then treat her accordingly. If he does not do so, the client may end up taking medication for many different symptoms, which is unnecessary, if not counterproductive. There may also be an internal part that is not willing to follow treatment recommendations due to beliefs about medication or what it means to get well. In such a case, it is important for the client to address the issue with her therapist.

A second reason for a psychiatrist to be aware of the DID diagnosis is that some medications can trigger dissociation or mimic dissociation. It is nonproductive to take medications that will magnify symptoms the client is already experiencing. It can also be retraumatizing for younger parts and can create unnecessary internal distress.

Doctors need to be aware that patients with DID may dissociate during sessions, which can create difficulties with medication compliance. This can be avoided by the client making sure that an adult part is out during the appointment and by writing things down or asking for written instructions. Most pharmacies provide patients with written information about the medication they are prescribed. If not, the client can certainly ask for it. If a client does dissociate and realizes later that he has some questions, it is perfectly appropriate to call the doctor and ask for clarification. Typically, a nurse will be able to talk with the patient and explain things. If not, doctors are usually willing to return calls. Do not expect an immediate callback, however. Because doctors are generally on busy schedules, it is often best to leave a specific message and a voice mail, E-mail, or fax that the doctor can use to get back to you. This method will save both time and aggravation in terms of having to wait for a return call.

On the first visit, the psychiatrist will probably ask about suicidal thoughts or past attempts. If not, the client needs to take responsibility for providing the doctor with that information so that any drugs prescribed will minimize the possibility of a fatal overdose. This information is especially important if a person is severely depressed or has problems with impulse control. Finally, clients must be aware that the doctor does not have the power to "fix" them; that may be magical thinking on their part. Clients need to be willing to be active participants with the treatment team, which means talking honestly with the therapist and psychiatrist, giving input as to their own goals regarding therapy, and asking for clarification when they are unsure about decisions being made regarding their treatment.

MEDICATION

Let's now look at some of the medications commonly used with DID clients and the symptoms they can be expected to target.[1] Depression and anxiety are typical diagnoses that accompany DID. In fact, a first encounter with a DID client often centers on a discussion of the depressive symptoms being presented. These symptoms include low mood, changes in appetite, sleep disturbances, difficulty concentrating or making decisions, fatigue, isolation, and in some cases, suicidal thoughts or actions. Major depression is more severe and is diagnosed when someone has been experiencing symptoms like the ones listed above, nearly every day, for at least two weeks. Dysthymia, another form of depression, is usually less severe in intensity but has been experienced by the person for at least two years. Dysthymia is comparable to having a low-grade fever that interferes with a person's ability to function yet she just cannot seem to shake it, whereas major depression is like having a sudden onset of a severe case of the flu. There are other diagnostic categories for depression as well. If someone believes she is depressed, it is important for her to seek help from a mental health professional. She might also want to read books on the subject, such as *The Depression Sourcebook* by Brian Quinn.

If a therapist recommends a psychiatric consultation because he believes a client is depressed, the client might be given a prescription for an antidepressant. The purpose of an antidepressant is to correct the imbalances in brain chemistry that create depression. It usually takes several weeks to notice a major difference in mood after starting an antidepressant, so it is important not to become discouraged and stop the medication too soon. It is equally important to talk with the doctor if there are any concerns about the medication's effectiveness.

DEPRESSION

The most typical medications prescribed for depression are *selective serotonin reuptake inhibitors* (SSRIs). These medications block the absorption of serotonin, a neurotransmitter in the brain, back into the cells that produced it. Serotonin is responsible for influencing a variety of functions, such as learning, sleep, and moods. Decreased levels of serotonin cannot lead only to depression, but may also point to an increased risk for suicide. Prozac is the SSRI with which most people are familiar. Paxil, Luvox, Celexa, and Zoloft are other commonly prescribed drugs in this category of antidepressants. These drugs are often used in an attempt to decrease suicidal thoughts. SSRIs can be used for atypical depression, a depression that does not fit the usual diagnostic categories in terms of types or severity of symptoms according to the *DSM-IV.* Although this is rare, some people actually become more anxious and agitated when taking these drugs. If this type of paradoxical reaction is experienced, it is important to call a doctor.

SSRIs are often prescribed for agitated depression, a depression that also includes symptoms such as anxiety or increased irritability or agitation. Approximately 80 percent of individuals suffering from depression also report some symptoms of anxiety, including unrealistic fears, agitation, irritability, or panic attacks. About 20 percent report increased feelings of agitation, 17 percent report generalized anxiety, and 10 percent suffer panic attacks in conjunction with depressive symptoms.[2] SSRIs can also be effective in the treatment of other disorders, such as obsessive-compulsive disorder, panic disorders, bulimia, and PTSD. Some of the more common side effects associated with these medications include nausea, diarrhea, sleepiness, and insomnia. On occasion, these drugs can cause tremors, restlessness, muscle spasms, and sexual dysfunction. It is important to keep in mind that not everyone experiences side effects, and the more severe side effects tend to be rare. If a person has questions or concerns about her medication, she should contact her doctor or pharmacist.

Some of the newer antidepressants commonly prescribed for depression are Effexor, Wellbutrin, Remeron, and Serzone. Effexor is often used to treat severe depression. It not only blocks the reuptake of serotonin, but also of norepinephrine (another brain neurotransmitter). The side effects of these antidepressants are similar to the ones associated with the SSRIs. A person might also experience dry mouth or constipation with Effexor or, in rare cases, an increase in blood pressure.

Wellbutrin works well for atypical or bipolar disorders. It has also been prescribed for people with attention deficit disorder. It is thought that Wellbutrin affects levels of dopamine and norepinephrine. In some cases, people experience agitation or insomnia when taking Wellbutrin. Consequently, it is not recommended for people with agitated depression. It is also not recommended for people with eating disorders or seizure disorders, which is important to keep in mind when treating DID patients. It is not at all unusual for a diagnosis of DID and eating disorder to coexist, although the eating disorder may be confined to a particular alter.

Serzone also blocks the reuptake of serotonin and can be very helpful in treating anxiety and the sleep disturbances often associated with depression. Common side effects include dizziness and possibly feeling overly sedated throughout the day. Serzone is also used at times in the treatment of fibromyalgia and migraines, two common complaints of female trauma survivors. Many of the headaches associated with DID, however, are related to dissociation and switching behavior. It is important to discuss that possibility with a doctor.

The *tricyclic antidepressants* are also used to treat depression, but they tend to have greater side effects, including dry mouth, blurred vision, dizziness, sexual dysfunction, weight gain, and a higher risk of overdose. In societies in which thinness is overly emphasized, many patients refuse to take medications that might cause weight gain. In addition, in the case of eating disorders, weight gain could trigger symptoms. Tricyclics, however, are sometimes prescribed for bulimia as a way of decreasing urges. The tricyclics work by inhibiting the absorption of neurotransmitters back into the cells that produced them. These drugs are often successful in the treatment of chronic pain, another complaint among many trauma survivors.

It is important for a client's therapist and psychiatrist to work closely together whenever possible. Many of the physical complaints associated with DID are *psychogenic* in nature, meaning that they are caused by emotional stress. Others are very clearly the result of brain alterations associated with PTSD. It is not easy to determine which is which, and the two are so interrelated that a chicken and egg scenario is created. Thus, good communication among health care providers is important, and being treated from a holistic perspective is usually more effective than treating individual symptoms.

A final class of antidepressants is the *monoamine oxidase inhibitors (MAOIs)*. These drugs work by preventing the breaking down of serotonin and norepinephrine, neurotransmitters in the brain that are responsible for regulating mood. These drugs also prevent the breakdown of tyramine, however, so eating foods that are high in tyramine, such as cheese and red wine, can increase blood pressure to dangerously high levels. Other less serious side effects include drowsiness, dry mouth, constipation, and drops in blood pressure when standing too quickly.

MAOIs are rarely prescribed as a first line of defense in the treatment of depression due to the stringent dietary guidelines. A patient can also suffer adverse effects when combining these drugs with other medications, which is important to consider when treating DID. If there is not good communication and cooperation among internal parts, it could be dangerous to prescribe these drugs to DID clients.

Typically, MAOIs are prescribed when a person does not respond to other medications. They are also used for atypical depression and bipolar disorder and can be effective for treating panic, social phobia, and PTSD. Other options for treating these disorders are available, however, and if it is possible to find a medication that has fewer side effects and still decreases symptoms, that may be the more appropriate choice. If a doctor suggests MAOIs and the client has any concerns about his ability to follow the diet restrictions, it is important to discuss that issue with the doctor.

ANXIETY

Anxiety is another disorder often experienced by individuals with DID, which is not surprising considering that PTSD is classified as an anxiety disorder. Benzodiazepines are often prescribed for mild anxiety because they are fast acting and can be taken as needed. This class of medications includes such drugs as Ativan, Xanax, Klonopin, Valium, Librium, and Tranxene. Side effects include sedation, fatigue, drowsiness, and possible disorientation. Abuse of these drugs can lead to dependency, and they should not be used with alcohol because that can increase the sedative effect to dangerous levels. In fact, the use of benzodiazepines with alcohol or barbiturates can be lethal.

Discontinuing use of these medications needs to be done under a doctor's supervision to avoid withdrawal, symptoms of which can include insomnia, agitation, anxiety, and, in more severe cases, seizures and coma. If these medications are taken as prescribed, however, they can be very helpful for managing anxiety, including panic attacks and mania.

BuSpar is another commonly prescribed drug that is helpful for anxiety. It is also safe to use for people who are chemically dependent and who may be unable to use the faster-acting benzodiazepines. BuSpar can also be used in conjunction with antidepressants. Common side effects include headaches, stomachaches, dizziness, and fatigue.

Other medications used for anxiety are certain antihistamines such as Atarax, Vistaril, and Benadryl. These drugs also tend to be safer for use by people who have a history of chemical abuse. Beta-blockers, which are antihypertensive drugs normally thought of in terms of their use with cardiovascular diseases, are also employed at times to treat anxiety. Beta-blockers work by blocking the effects of adrenaline in the body's beta-receptors. This blocking is important when treating anxiety disorders because when the body is flooded with adrenaline, it remains in a constant state of fight or flight, the biological protection device that keeps us alert and prepared to flee danger. Such a state also produces symptoms most commonly associated with anxiety disorders. Inderal, a commonly used beta-blocker, can be utilized to treat performance anxiety. These drugs are often used to treat migraine headaches as well. Side effects include dizziness, hypotension, and brachycardia (decreased heart rate).

Many different mood stabilizers can be helpful in treating the anxiety and affective dysregulation that often accompanies trauma disorders. Depakote, Lithium, Tegretol, and Neurontin are also used to treat severe anxiety or agitation.

The final class of medications useful for persons with DID is the neuroleptics, which block receptors for the neurotransmitter dopamine. Trilafon and Haldol are often prescribed to treat flashbacks, and Mellaril is a drug that can be prescribed for the purpose of sedation with severe anxiety or agitation. Newer and safer drugs, such as Risperdal, Zyrexa, and Seroquel, are used for the intrusive symptoms associated with PTSD and can be helpful in terms of their sedative effect and ability to induce a state of relaxation. These drugs are not routinely prescribed and, in less severe cases of anxiety, an antianxiety drug such as BuSpar or a minor tranquilizer will be effective in managing symptoms. Naltrexone has been shown to reduce dissociative symptoms and flashbacks for some patients. In one study, patients reported "a highly significant reduction" in the intensity and duration of dissociative phenomena and a "significant reduction" in the number of flashbacks after at least three days of taking the medication.[3] (See Table 7.1.)

ALTERNATIVE TREATMENTS

Some patients are adamantly opposed to taking medications, although their reasons may vary. Some natural remedies can be used for depression, anxiety, and sleep; some of the most commonly used are briefly mentioned here.

Warning: Do not self-medicate, even when using herbal remedies. Instead, find a doctor who is willing to discuss both traditional and alternative methods of treatment and then work together to form the treatment plan that will be most helpful.

Table 7.1 Common Medications Used in the Treatment of Depression and Anxiety

DEPRESSION:

Medication	Severe	Bipolar	Atypical	With Anxiety and Insomnia	With Panic
Tricyclics	X			X	
Effexor	X				
SRIs	X	X	X		X
Wellbutrin		X			
MAOIs		X	X		
Lithium		X			
Paxil				X	
Serzone				X	
Remaron				X	
Trazodone				X	
Benzodiazepines					X

As discussed previously, trauma survivors tend to share several issues, including bouts with depression, anxiety, insomnia, and acute stress reactions that may include flashbacks or hypervigilance and arousal. Some of the most common alternative methods of treatment for these symptoms are listed below.

St.-John's-Wort

Many people suffering from depression are turning to St.-John's-wort instead of more popular antidepressants such as Prozac and Zoloft. This wildflower has been used for years in Europe and is

Table 7.1 Common Medications Used in the Treatment of Depression and Anxiety, *continued*

ANXIETY:

Medication	PTSD	Generalized Anxiety	OCD	Panic	With Depression and Insomnia
Luvox	X		X		
Naltrexone	X				
Benzodiazepines		X		X	
BuSpar		X			
Beta-blockers, such as Inderal		X			
Antihistamines, such as Atarax and Vistaril		X			
Effexor		X			
Prozac			X		
Paxil			X		X
Zoloft			X		
Celexa			X		
Anafran			X		
SSRIs				X	
Tricyclics				X	
Serzone					X
Remeron					X
Trazodone					X

approved in Germany for the treatment of depression and anxiety. St.-John's-wort relieves insomnia and anxiety, improves appetite, diminishes fatigue, increases a general sense of physical well-being, elevates mood, and decreases feelings of emotional vulnerability.[4] It is not known exactly how St.-John's-wort works, but it may be in the same way that the SSRIs do, by helping regulate levels of the neurotransmitters serotonin and norepinephrine. It has been suggested that St.-John's-wort has similar properties to the MAOIs. Consequently, a person may need to follow the MAOI dietary guidelines when taking this herb. It is best to talk to a doctor about whether that diet is necessary.

S-Adenosyl-L-Methionine

S-adenosyl-L-methionine (SAM-e) has been found to relieve symptoms of depression. It produces the neurotransmitters serotonin, dopamine, norepinephrine, and epinephrine, which are all needed to maintain normal mood levels.

Kava

Kava is an herb that grows on the islands of the South Pacific. It is used primarily for treating anxiety. Many people also find it helpful in managing the insomnia that often accompanies depression and anxiety. Kava is able to relieve anxiety without the sedating effect of tranquilizers. Although it may not be as effective for severe or chronic anxiety, kava does seem to be adequate for milder anxiety associated with daily stress.

Chamomile

Another herb used for decreasing anxiety is chamomile, which is often taken in tea before bedtime. It has been used for years to calm restlessness or nervousness and is readily available in many forms, including capsules, teas, and tinctures. Bathing in chamomile is also a good way to calm the mind and body in preparation for sleep.

Lavender

Lavender can be added to bath water or lavender candles can be paired with soothing music as a way to induce relaxation. It helps to ease headaches as well, and the aroma of lavender is comforting to most people.

Valerian

Valerian is another herb that helps induce sleep without the nasty side effects of tranquilizers or other sleep medications. This plant is used for restlessness and poor sleep from pain or trauma; it acts upon the central nervous system as a depressant.[5]

Homeopathy

Homeopathy was founded by a German physician, Samuel Hahnemann, in the late 1700s and is based on the belief that "like cures like." Substances that create certain symptoms in healthy people are thought to cure the same symptoms in someone who is ill. Therefore, if someone is ill with a virus, the remedy includes highly diluted elements of the virus itself. Homeopathic remedies can also be useful in treating the symptoms associated with acute or chronic stress. These remedies can be obtained through a homeopathic practitioner or in most natural health food stores. They are easy to use and do not produce the side effects commonly associated with traditional medications or even some herbs.

Flower Essences

Flower essences tend to be less well known to the general public than other alternative treatments, but they can also be used for a variety of physical and emotional complaints. Flower essences are based on the work of bacteriologist Edward Bach. Robert Stevens, an instructor at the New Mexico School of Natural Therapeutics, describes flower essences as "resonance," energy in a state of vibrational movement.[6] Bach flower practitioners believe in treating the body and mind in unity. One particular remedy, Rescue Remedy, is a combination of flower essences used to treat the shock, panic, and dissociation that arises in emergency situations. Proponents of flower essences carry Rescue Remedy with them and use a few drops under the tongue whenever they experience extreme stress.

SUMMARY

The list of medications and alternative treatments mentioned here is by no means exhaustive, but simply serves as a brief introduction into the use of drugs, herbs, homeopathic remedies, and flower essences. If any of the alternative treatments seems viable to a person with DID, she can talk with someone who has specific training in alternative medicine or her own doctor. Alternative does not automatically mean safe, and it may be dangerous to mix some herbs with medications that are being taken. A doctor or pharmacist can clarify those issues.

Because we are complex beings, a pill, regardless of its form, is rarely enough to create a cure. In addition to psychotherapy, individuals can take charge of their own healing by finding the path that is right for them. Meditation, yoga, prayer, and imagery are all valuable tools for changing negative thought patterns and managing anxiety more effectively. Immersing one's self in the practice of a spiritual path will promote an overall sense of well-being, which helps to stimulate the healing process. Healing is as individual as the person who is seeking relief. Belief in an ability to effect change is probably the most valuable tool available.

FAQS ABOUT
MEDICATION AND DID

Q Why do I have to take medication at all? Shouldn't therapy be enough?

A Many people think therapy should be enough, and sometimes it is, but persons with DID often have other diagnoses, including depression and anxiety. Others may have a diagnosis of PTSD in addition to DID. These people might experience flashbacks and sleep disorders. These symptoms are often biologically based and respond best to medication. The medication helps decrease symptoms to a level where therapy can then be effective. Trauma affects brain functioning, but exactly how this occurs is unknown. Harvard researcher Bessel van der Kolk conducts extensive research in the area of trauma and its effects on the brain. As research continues and the relationship between trauma and brain functioning is better understood, the implications of that research on the treatment of DID will be phenomenal.

Q Will I have to be on medication the rest of my life?

A It is important to discuss with your doctor the length of time you will be on medication if it concerns you. Most people take medication until symptoms subside and then slowly decrease the dosage under their doctors' supervision. Others take medication throughout their lives, but only when symptoms reappear. Yet others may have to take medication at a maintenance level throughout their lives. It depends on the person and the symptoms being treated. It is helpful to think of the symptoms associated with trauma in the same way as an illness like diabetes; rarely do people refuse to take their insulin because they know how important it is to their continued health. The same is true of medications prescribed for psychological disorders.

Q I am in recovery. Can medications cause me to relapse?

A This question is one for which getting an answer is important. Be sure to tell your doctor that you are chemically dependent and ask for a medication that is nonaddictive. Benzodiazepines, which are often prescribed for the anxiety that is associated with PTSD, can be harmful to people with addictions. Do not avoid medications because you are chemically dependent, however. Many nonaddictive medications are available. It is not necessary for you to suffer needlessly.

Q Why do I have to take medication when it is another part that is anxious?

A DID is the way an individual experiences life. In reality, though, you are still one person in one body. If your doctor could take all your internal parts, with all their symptoms, and bring them into a unified consciousness, you would see that the anxiety one alter holds is also a part of you. When treating DID, it is important for the doctor to be able to treat you as a unified person. Cooperation and communication among internal parts is an integral step toward healing.

Q Is it normal for people with DID to have difficulty sleeping? I never seem to feel rested, even though I go to bed at a reasonable hour each night.

A Moshe Torem discovered a subgroup of patients diagnosed with DID and sleep apnea. Treating the apnea reduced dissociative switching and amnesia during the day.[7] Another possible reason for not feeling rested is the hypervigilance associated with PTSD, which may mean that you are on alert, so to speak, even in your sleep. Some DID patients even report alter activity during the night, which is obviously going to have an effect on the body. If lack of sleep begins to affect your ability to function during the day, ask your doctor for something to help you sleep. Also take advantage of herbal teas, warm baths, and soothing music as a part of your bedtime routine.

Chapter Eight

Learning to Trust Again: The Group Therapy Process

Chris had been in therapy for dissociative identity disorder for one year. Now his therapist was suggesting group therapy. "Why?" he asked. "I like coming here and I am doing well." The therapist smiled and readily agreed with the assessment that Chris was making regarding his own therapy. Then he added, "Chris, my suggestion to begin group therapy is not about ending your therapy here. And it is certainly not about a belief on my part that our work together is not helpful. It is about sharing your story with other people who have experienced trauma." Chris took a deep breath, but said nothing for several seconds. Finally, he asked thoughtfully, "What exactly, is the goal if I decide to attend a group?"

"The goal" answered the therapist, "is to share your story with people who truly understand so that you can experience their support as you work through your own feelings of distrust and shame. It is also about continuing to learn skills that will help you live more successfully in the here and now. I am not saying that cannot happen here, but I do believe you gain something much deeper when you become a part of a group. Think about it and we'll discuss the idea more in the weeks to come."

Most clients react with uncertainty when confronted with suggestions to begin group therapy. For some, it is simply a question of whether group therapy is really necessary. For others, the reaction is one of extreme anxiety often based on the misbelief that the therapist is trying to "get rid of them." Even mental health professionals react with differing positions and thoughts about the appropriateness of group therapy for DID clients. This chapter discusses the various types of groups and when it might be helpful for a DID client to attend one. Ultimately, the decision will lie with the therapist and client based on, for example, the amount of time an individual has been in therapy, therapy goals, and whether a particular group is a fit for them.

SUPPORT GROUPS

There are different types of groups that a person might attend. Support groups are usually just that: for support. They are rarely led by therapists, although some are. Formats may differ, but the basic goal of a group is for people with similar issues to come together to share and receive support. The best-known support groups are the twelve-step groups based on the twelve steps of Alcoholics Anonymous (AA). Twelve-step groups exist for many issues, including overeating, managing emotions, and codependency. Some people with DID have also attended Alcoholics Anonymous or Narcotics Anonymous to deal with their own addictions.

Addictions—be they to alcohol, pain medication, or food—are often a part of a dissociative disorder. Addictions may develop as a person attempts to medicate painful emotions. They are also a way of regulating the intrusive symptoms associated with PTSD. For others, addictions may develop due to the acting-out behavior related to a particular emotional state, such as anger. Regardless of why the addiction is there, dissociators might find themselves in a meeting similar to AA. Alcoholics Anonymous is a highly successful program for treating alcoholism. Anyone with a desire to stop drinking can call the general AA number listed in the telephone book and ask for a list of meetings in her area. For someone with DID, it can be helpful to attend a meeting that is for persons with emotional disorders as well as addictions. If it feels too frightening to go to a meeting alone, he can request that someone from the group give him a call and then meet him there. Another possibility is to attend a speaker meeting where people go to hear someone else talk about her own addiction, giving newcomers the opportunity to sit back and learn about the AA program. One helpful thing about twelve-step programs is that they provide the structure of meeting at the same time each week and the encouragement for people to find a sponsor who can offer them guidance in learning how to work the steps. AA groups differ in personality, so if one group does not work, it is important to try another.

AA, however, is not for everyone. Some people believe AA is for recovery from alcoholism only, and that following the steps is enough to accomplish that in every case. Consequently, some people may frown on the use of medication and may discourage any talk about emotional issues that might be affecting someone's addictions. Another aspect of AA groups that can cause difficulty for women is that this program was originally formed to help men who had tried everything else and failed. Some people in the groups can adopt a rather authoritarian and rigid approach to the way they believe people need to follow the program. To a dissociator, this attitude might feel very much like abusive relationships they have had in the past, so for some people, the dynamics can be triggering. For someone with DID, it is important for an adult part to attend the meetings. If a younger part operates more like a teen, yet feels that she shares the addiction, she can share space with the adult. Such sharing helps increase co-consciousness and decrease the likelihood of being triggered. It is helpful to remember that all the parts together create the whole person.

One group that has had success with women with addictions is Women for Sobriety. The group's philosophy is to "forget the past, plan for tomorrow, and live for today." This philosophy is good for trauma survivors as well, although dissociators should be encouraged to accept and integrate the past as opposed to forgetting it. Another successful support group for women is Sixteen Steps for Personal Empowerment. This group focuses on the needs of many women to increase self-esteem and personal empowerment as a part of their recovery process. For some women, these groups feel emotionally safer than other groups because the format is less rigid and the emphasis is on empowerment rather than powerlessness. If a past abuser was male, certain dynamics in AA could be triggering, but that is not an excuse for not dealing with an addiction. Instead, it is important to seek out a women's group within the AA program or a program such as those mentioned above.

Other types of support groups have a facilitator, often someone with a good amount of recovery time, who coordinates meetings. I once cofacilitated an adult attention deficit disorder (ADD) group with someone who had ADD. The group format consisted of a specific educational topic that was presented each week, followed by time for group discussion. Groups such as this one can be formed for virtually anything, given the interest. Some support groups are run entirely by members of the group, but outside speakers are invited to present and then group members meet to talk. Some eating disorder groups also use this format. Once again, to benefit most from the group, it is important for an adult part to be present. It is also important to recognize that regardless of the particular format, these groups exist to provide support. An individual needs to be far enough along in therapy that she is able to listen to the opinions of others without feeling as if she automatically must make them her own. If a client does not have the ability to do that at least to some extent, it is helpful for her to talk with her therapist about the appropriateness of attending a support group.

PSYCHOEDUCATIONAL GROUPS

Another type of group is the psychoeducational group. These groups are similar to support groups, but are usually more structured, are typically run by a therapist or other professional person, and are often limited in time. Psychoeducational groups can be a good starting point because clients can gain information about DID, trauma, and coping techniques without having to share a lot of in-depth information about themselves. The goal of these groups is usually living more effectively in the here and now, and they offer helpful information that can be discussed further in individual therapy. DBT groups, explained more fully in chapter 6, are an example of this type of group. DBT groups are extremely structured. A typical group provides a brief check-in time regarding the skills being practiced. The bulk of the group time includes education about effective communication skills and the management of emotions. Each group concludes with a plan for practicing newly learned skill, as well as reinforcing skills already learned.

THERAPY GROUPS

The therapy group is the topic of the rest of this chapter. Trained therapists lead therapy groups. Some are time limited, which means that they meet for a specified number of weeks and then the group ends. Others are open ended and run indefinitely. If a client has been in therapy long enough to have worked through most of her memory issues, her therapist might recommend a specific type of therapy group as an adjunct to individual therapy, such as a women's issues group, an anger management group, or a group for anxiety management. Regardless of where a person is in therapy, her individual therapist might recommend a DID or trauma-focused therapy group.

Typically, these groups provide the opportunity for members to process the various issues associated with DID, such as shame, trust, fear of abandonment, and learning to manage daily stress. The list is endless. Of course, the biggest benefit of a therapy group is the opportunity to be with other people who are DID and understand what it is like to live with the disorder. It can help a person feel less alone. It also affords group members the opportunity to talk openly about their dissociation without fear of reprisal. Therapists who oppose DID groups generally do so based on the belief that these groups keep people stuck in the disorder. In other words, if dissociators surround themselves with other people who are DID, they might become so accepting of each other and the use of dissociation and switching behaviors that they will not feel a need to move beyond those defenses. Those arguments, however, are not usually heard in regard to other types of therapy groups, such as those for anxiety management or chemical dependency, and some therapists disagree with that view, provided the group facilitator is experienced in treating DID and understands the importance of teaching dissociators to live in the present.

Another concern among therapists is the fear of contamination among group members. Dissociators are often from family systems with poor boundaries and also tend to operate, at times, in trance states that can leave them highly impressionable. The concern is that hearing stories of group members' past abuse might overly influence some individuals. They might begin to adopt some of those memories as their own or, at the very least, become triggered by what others share.

A third concern is that clients with borderline traits might get into competition with other group members about who has the most sensational abuse stories or who can get the most attention from the therapist, which can keep them stuck in the past or stuck in behaviors that are unhealthy. These behaviors are not limited to DID groups, by the way, but the very nature of the psychological injury experienced by those with DID certainly sets the stage for these dynamics to be more prominent in a DID group. To be able to address these issues in a group setting could be a valuable experience, though.

All these concerns are valid and have to do with developmental deficits that result from childhood trauma, but these issues can be addressed at the onset of the group. A solution is for DID therapy groups to be facilitated by a therapist who has experience in treating DID and who is able to set very clear goals and boundaries regarding the purpose and structure of the group. Good, responsible treatment of DID must focus on helping clients to develop coping skills that will help them to manage current stressors and live in the here and now, with an eventual decrease in the amount of switching, self-injurious behavior, and the overall use of dissociation as a defense. Too much emphasis on the past can keep a person unnecessarily stuck and can put her in a role where she feels so emotionally dependent that she is unable to meet her own needs effectively.

Another solution is to run a trauma group, as opposed to one that is specifically for clients with DID, because therapists who treat DID are actually treating trauma issues. A trauma group will address issues shared by clients with many different diagnoses, including PTSD, DID, BPD, and DDNOS. The mix of diagnoses can actually help group members focus on the management of their trauma symptoms rather than attaching a lot of meaning to a particular diagnosis, which tends to be more productive in the long run. A trauma approach to therapy acknowledges that it is trauma, in general, that leads to dissociation, as opposed to one particular experience that is shared by all dissociators.

Some of the advantages of group therapy are subtle. For example, a person can benefit just by listening to others. Or, as group members share, they might begin to view their own issues differently. They might also begin to see how, as human beings, we have much in common. It can be comforting to realize that other people face similar challenges, have the same emotions we do, and have learned to cope. If a client is in an open group, she will have the benefit of seeing others who have been a part of the group for much longer and have probably reached a growth point that she has only imagined until now. These people provide hope simply by being present. In addition, as clients begin to open up and relate to others more genuinely, they will begin to experience an increased acceptance of both self and others.

If a client is involved in both individual and group therapy, the group experience can also help her to learn to expand her relationships beyond the scope of the relationships she has developed with her individual therapist. This can be difficult if someone has DID because expanding the support network can trigger the same trust and abandonment issues for a client that could occur if she were forced to leave therapy prematurely. Consciously making that choice, however, gives a person an excellent opportunity to confront her fears, knowing there is a safety net below. This kind of healthy experimentation leads to growth. It is the same sort of process that children go through at various developmental stages. In healthy families, the parents are like the supportive therapist who encourages the client to step out into the unknown, yet welcomes her back at any time. The foray into the group process is most certainly a step into the unknown, but this strange land will soon begin to feel like home. As group members come and go, valuable lessons will be learned about acceptance and letting go, necessary skills in every relationship. Relationships end, even good ones, and there is grief that accompanies those losses. The therapy group can provide a safe place to explore those losses.

THE GROUP PROCESS

Although various types of groups have been discussed, it is also important to consider how groups work. I. D. Yalom has studied the effectiveness of group therapy throughout the years and has observed that people heal due, in part, to what he refers to as curative factors. He lists several important factors, ranging from group cohesiveness to various interpersonal factors, that occur as relationships develop within the group.[1] Part of what occurs for group members is the gaining of hope that things truly can change for the better, along with the understanding that no one is completely alone in his suffering. It is a part of the human condition. This realization allows group members to begin to share more of themselves, without feeling threatened or alienated. The group experience also teaches members that they can give to others in the midst of their own pain. The experience of offering reassurance or a listening ear to someone else has a way of decreasing the intense preoccupation that many people have in regard to their own suffering. Becoming a member of a group can teach a person simply how to "be" with others. This socialization process, which eventually leads to a deeper level of intimacy, is helpful for dissociators who have put a lot of energy into being separate from self and others.

It is not just the type of group that a person attends that matters, but the group dynamics that are involved as well. In group therapy, members tend to exhibit the same behavioral patterns that they do with other people in their lives, behaviors that originated in childhood. The group provides a valuable learning experience as well as a place to begin practicing new behaviors. In fact, it helps to think of the group as a learning lab that will provide its members with insights about themselves and the way they relate to others. Fortunately, labs are created for experimentation. So, in a client's personal group therapy lab, she gets the opportunity to experiment week after week. The following are a few experiments with which to begin. Group members can:

- Take the risk of sharing something about themselves, however small, at every session.
- Practice giving feedback to others in the group.
- Allow themselves to be genuine with at least one emotion they normally avoid.
- Practice accepting feedback from others in the group without becoming defensive or switching.
- When feeling angry or uncomfortable, practice taking ownership of their thoughts and feelings and share them with the group.

If you are a dissociator who is attending a group or considering attending one, add some things of your own you would like to try out in the lab. Think of yourself as the Marie Curie of the group therapy learning lab. Your goal: self-discovery!

THE THERAPIST/FACILITATOR ROLE

A freely interactive group, with few structural restrictions, will, in time, develop into a social microcosm of the participant members. (Yalom, 1985)

This statement is true, even if applied to a more specialized group such as one for individuals with DID. Yet DID groups will certainly come packaged with their own set of obstacles to overcome. The initial tasks for the therapists remain the same, however. A therapist will have to think about how to create an appropriate group, establish boundaries that will be helpful to the members, and most important, address the here and now with a client population that is, for the most part, terrified of living in the present.

Creating an appropriate group in terms of membership has much more attached to it than making sure prospective members have a diagnosis of DID. It involves assessing the client's goals to see if they are complementary to those of the group facilitators. Also involved is a discussion between the client's primary therapist and the group therapist so that the latter can better understand the client's ability to stay in the present, contain powerful emotional material, and both contribute and receive feedback from other group members. The group therapist will also want to know that the client has done enough memory work to be able to focus on present coping and interpersonal skills. An important question for the referring therapist is why she is making the referral now. If the answer is simply that the therapist is feeling overwhelmed herself, that is probably not the most appropriate reason for a group referral. If the group therapist and individual therapist can formulate goals that complement each other and benefit the client, however, the referral will probably be a success. There is nothing unusual about an individual therapist feeling overwhelmed in the course of treatment, and bringing in another therapist can often be helpful.

The establishment of group boundaries will include things common to all groups, such as confidentiality and attending sessions on time. In a DID group, though, it will also be necessary to address whether switching is allowed, whether discussion of past abuse is allowed, and so on. These issues must be addressed initially to avoid unnecessary conflicts in the future should a client feel abandoned or betrayed because she is not allowed to discuss certain issues or behave in certain ways.

The facilitator also needs to recognize that even if past issues are brought to the group, the here and now focus continues to be of primary importance. In other words, he must be willing to address group process in addition to content. If not, facilitating a DID group is not advisable because working with process, at some level, is essential. When facilitating a DID group, the therapist is dealing with many diagnoses in addition to the primary diagnosis of DID. Group members may be dealing with depression, anxiety, addictions, borderline traits, or PTSD. The interpersonal dynamics will be experienced on both an internal and external level as well. The combination of individual and group dynamics can become quite complicated, and it will be up to the facilitator to help the group members to process both the content and the relational issues that come to play in any given session. Such a process involves a lot of skill and attention, which is why DID groups are best facilitated by cotherapists.

Yalom describes various group stages, beginning with the initial stage, in which group members experience orientation and hesitation about the group process, initial and increased participation in the process, search for meaning, and emotional dependency. Then comes the second stage, which focuses more on relational issues that occur in the form of conflict, domination, and rebellion. This stage in turn leads to the third stage, which focuses on the development of group cohesiveness.

The attributes inherent in these stages mirror much of what is encountered by DID clients in nearly every relationship in which they participate. Consequently, therapists need to be experienced in the treatment of DID before attempting to become a cotherapist for a group.

Group therapists are most likely to experience success if they:

1. Understand the treatment of DID.
2. Cofacilitate a group with a therapist they know well and who shares their theoretical orientation.

3. Have clearly defined the goals and boundaries of the group.
4. Have talked with each prospective member's therapist regarding his goals for the client and the ability of the client to succeed in a group therapy format.
5. Have conducted a pretherapy interview with each client to discuss therapy goals, to discuss beliefs about the capacity to be an active group participant, and to rule out any severe pathology that would impede the ability to succeed in a group setting.
6. Seek ongoing supervision in the treatment of DID or group therapy facilitation if they do not have an adequate level of experience or expertise in these areas.

Group therapy can be a powerful addition to individual work being done, but it is important for therapists to suggest it at a time when they believe it will be most advantageous for the client. When working with a DID client, the first step is stabilization. That is not the time to introduce group work, because it is likely to be too overwhelming. The initial goal is to develop rapport with the client and help her to learn containment skills so that self-injurious behaviors can be managed. This time is also when both the therapist and the client begin to gain an understanding of how the client's internal system operates. Only after this point should a therapy group be considered. Trauma work follows this initial stage of therapy. Whether someone should attend a group in the midst of trauma work depends on the type of group being contemplated. If the group is for DID clients, a therapist needs to consider the following:

1. Is there more than one therapist facilitating the group experienced in treating DID?
2. Does the group focus allow for the sharing of past trauma, and at what level?

In-depth sharing about past trauma is not generally advised in a group setting for DID clients.[2] If the referral seems appropriate, however, what becomes important is open communication between the individual and group therapists so splitting does not occur and salient information that is processed is addressed in both settings.

If the group focus is only on coping in the here and now, the majority of the trauma work will need to be done before making a referral. At the very least, the client will need to have a good understanding of her own dissociative process and enough co-consciousness to be able to stay in the present the majority of the time. It could be difficult for a client to attend a DID group that has an "absolutely no switching" rule. That stance is overly rigid for this client population and could be experienced as being punitive. Clear boundaries regarding group expectations, however, are essential.

BOUNDARIES

Some examples of group boundaries include the following, depending on the group:

1. Confidentiality is respected; whatever is shared in the group session stays there.
2. Past trauma will be discussed generally so as not to create undue stress for other group members. No graphic descriptions of past trauma are allowed.
3. Group members will not leave a session without alerting one of the facilitators about where they are going. This rule will help to ensure the safety of all members.
4. Respect will be shown to other group members. Abusive language directed at others will not be allowed.
5. Touching other group members is allowed only with the

permission of that person. For example, a group member might ask, "Can I give you a hug?" but must then wait for a response from the other person.

TREATMENT TECHNIQUES

A therapist can use many different techniques within the context of one group. Choice will have to do with the personality of the group at any given time, goals of the group, and therapist expertise. If the group is psychoeducational in nature, the therapist will probably want to present the educational piece, allow time for discussion, and then assign homework so that group participants can practice skills. For example, one group session might be devoted to learning how to manage anxiety. The therapist could first present information about the causes and types of anxiety. Then, after a discussion of how anxiety is experienced by various group members, the therapist could teach breathing techniques, basic mindfulness meditation, and imagery. She would then assign a specific skill, such as practicing calming breathing three times a day, for group members to practice until the next session.

If the group is more process oriented, with focus on learning coping skills to use in the here and now, the facilitator can expect to do a lot of redirecting. The therapist might allow group members to help each other determine appropriate coping techniques for situations that are presented. The therapy group that allows for processing of trauma will need a therapist, preferably cotherapists, who are able to help clients with the containment of strong emotional content.

There is room in each of the group settings for the use of creative techniques that can enhance the group experience. Experiential therapy that uses such techniques as art, writing, imagery, and relaxation is an example of a way in which group members can work individually or together to process emotions or synthesize newly learned material. Members might be encouraged to share their own poetry, journal writings, or collages to express the internal conflicts or victories that have been occurring. Or the facilitator can assign very specific projects for group members to work on during sessions. Although this book cannot begin to cover all the experiential therapy techniques possible, a few are given below. Clients who are easily triggered should not attempt to do these exercises on their own without first consulting their primary therapists.

Exercise 1

Goal For clients to begin to think about ways they can keep themselves grounded in the present.

Directions Have each group participant draw a clock or other measurement of time (calendar, hourglass, etc.) on a large piece of paper. Then title the page "Things that keep me grounded in (the present year)." Allow participants to write, draw, use symbols, or paste words and pictures from magazines that help them illustrate coping skills or relaxation activities that keep them grounded. Allow approximately thirty minutes for the activity and then let those who want to share do so.

Exercise 2

Goal For clients to identify internal strengths.

Directions Give each group member clay (and assorted craft objects, if desired), along with the instructions to make something from the clay that represents an aspect of their past trauma that they would like to overcome. Allow approximately twenty minutes. Then instruct the participants to take an additional piece of clay and mold something that will illustrate an internal trait that is more powerful than the past trauma or obstacle. Again allow approximately twenty minutes and then encourage people to share their work. The importance of the facilitator's role is to be able to encourage individuals regarding their ability to tap into internal strengths.

Exercise 3

Goal For clients to begin to identify healthy ways of nurturing themselves during both stressful and nonstressful times.
Directions Assign a group collage entitled "Healthy ways of nurturing myself." Allow thirty to forty minutes for group members to cut out words and pictures from magazines to put on the group collage that you then hang in the group room. The facilitator may need to offer assistance if group members are choosing unhealthy alternatives, such as smoking or drinking. They may also find that some participants will have a difficult time fully understanding the concept of self-nurturance. The facilitator can offer educational pieces and encouragement throughout the activity and then allow at least forty minutes for the group to process the experience.

Exercise 4

Goal To allow clients time to access internal thoughts and feelings of which they may not be consciously aware.
Directions Allow for a twenty-minute journal period to write on whatever topic seems appropriate for the group at the time. Writing can be especially useful at times when group members are stuck on an issue and the therapist needs to help create forward movement. It can also be used as a means of self-exploration. With a free-writing technique,

the instructions are very simple. The facilitator can either announce a topic, such as anger, or can give the first sentence of the writing, as in "I notice that I dissociate when . . . " Instruct participants to start writing and continue to do so until time is called. The facilitator must be sure to emphasize that it is important for the client to write whatever comes to mind, regardless of whether it makes sense, and to silence the inner critic or editor. In other words, participants should keep writing for the entire time without stopping to think or to make corrections. Then the facilitator will allow participants to share without comment from other group members. Because many DID clients tend to be shame based, it is very important for the facilitator to present this exercise in a nonthreatening, nonjudgmental manner, allowing people to pass during the sharing time if they so choose.

Exercise 5

Goal To create group cohesiveness while individuals access internal thoughts and feelings that may not be entirely conscious.

Directions The facilitator asks group members to write a group poem or story, with each person adding a line or more as they go around the circle. The facilitator can let the group choose a topic that is important to them collectively or assign a topic that she thinks will be beneficial, such as "Things I've learned through surviving trauma." When finished, participants will need time to read the finished project and process it as a group.

Art Therapy

Some groups are run specifically as art therapy groups. Common goals in these groups are for members to access internal emotions, further process trauma, or have an additional means of expression to complement work that is done through talk therapy. These groups need to be facilitated by a therapist with training in both art therapy and DID. Other groups, however, can certainly incorporate some of these exercises as part of their regular group process. If, as facilitator, you have never used art as therapy, some supervision from a professional certified in art therapy or teaming up with an art therapist as a cofacilitator for the group is recommended. It is amazing to see the movement that can occur with clients when they begin to access their own creativity. Julia Cameron, author of *The Artist's Way*, likens creativity to the work of God.[3] It can be a very liberating concept for DID clients who have sometimes been forced to stifle expressive parts of themselves in the name of survival.

Imagery Exercise

The primary therapist can also take a few minutes for some imagery work with clients regarding the issue of whether to attend a group. A dissociator might choose to do this exercise alone, but will probably gain more benefit from the exercise if a therapist is guiding the process and she is able to fully immerse herself in the imagery work. This exercise should not be done alone by anyone who might be easily triggered.

To do this exercise, the participant needs to make herself as comfortable as possible. Both feet need to be on the floor to help the person stay grounded. It is also important for an adult part to be present. Then a decision can be made as to whether other parts need to be present as well. Once the decision has been made and internal parts feel safe, it is appropriate to proceed as shown in Exhibit 8.1.

Discuss the client's experience and then ask the following questions: Is there a way to include at least some of these things in your own group experience? How might you begin to do that?

Exhibit 8.1 My Ideal Group (Therapist's Script)

Take three slow deep breaths. Each time you exhale, notice your body relaxing a bit more. Notice how you can breathe tension away. Notice any places where your body is continuing to hold on to tension. Breathe in and direct the breath to that place of tension. Allow the breath to massage the tension away. (Pause) Now imagine, for the next few minutes, that you are attending the first session of your new therapy group. Notice what the room is like: the colors, the temperature of the room, the furniture style and arrangement. (Pause) How many people are there? Where are they sitting? What do you notice about the other people in the room? Allow all your senses to respond. (Pause) What is the emotional atmosphere of the group? (Pause) Now, make any changes that you need to feel completely safe. (Pause) Good! Take another deep breath, exhaling any remaining tension. Now allow yourself to experience the ideal group session, whatever that might be. Notice everything about your experience. Include all five senses in the experience. (Wait three to five minutes) Now begin to bring all your attention back to this room. As you breathe, notice the energy that is running through your arms and legs. As I begin to count from ten to one, feel yourself becoming more and more alert.

Ten—nine—eight—awakening—seven—six—feeling the ground beneath your feet (therapist should begin to speak louder and more quickly)—five—four—three—eyes opening—two—fully awake, alert, and grounded!

Now, if you need to shake your hands and feet to get the circulation going, please do so. Then take the next ten minutes to write about what you just experienced. Be as specific as possible, and then we will discuss the exercise.

THOUGHT QUESTIONS

Following are some questions that will help both clients and therapists start thinking about whether group therapy should be pursued. It is helpful for both the client and the therapist to think about these questions before discussing them, because they may differ in the way they view certain things.

1. As a client, what benefit would you hope to receive by attending a therapy group? As a therapist, what benefit would you hope your client would receive by attending a group?

2. What containment skills do you, as a client, have that you can use in the event that another group member's story triggers you? As the therapist, what do you believe your client's containment skills are?

3. How do other parts feel about attending a group? How will you, as the client, make the final decision about whether to join a group? As a therapist, do you have a particular bias about how you believe the decision should be made as to whether your client attends a group?

4. What feelings do you have about your therapist suggesting a group? Have you shared your reactions? Why or why not? As the therapist, are you clear about your own reasons for suggesting a group for your client?

5. As a client, what fears do you have about attending a group? List each fear and discuss it with your therapist. As the therapist, what fears do you think your client might have about attending a group? Be prepared to address these fears openly and honestly. Recognize that individual fears may be associated with different ego states, which means there may be a developmental issue involved.

Chapter Nine

Self-Help and Coping Strategies

This chapter is written specifically for the person with DID or another dissociative disorder. If you are a significant person in the life of someone who is dissociative, this chapter can also help you understand more about the dissociative experience.

The call came at 11:00 one night as I was watching a movie with my husband. It was a friend. "Hi, it's Jamie. I found a therapist, but can I ask you something?" He then went on for almost an hour talking about his fears of probably losing yet another therapist, which would make three. He couldn't understand why therapists kept referring him on when all he wanted was for someone to help him. I agreed that it must be very frustrating, but also suggested that he might be switching states and not realizing it. Could he be portraying himself in a menacing fashion with which the therapists weren't prepared to deal? If so, it could mean that he had a very angry part that was being self-protective. He thought about my hypothesis, but wasn't very willing to accept it. "All I know," he said, "is that I was talking to my therapist on the phone and the next thing I knew there was blood all over." I could hear the terror in my friend's voice, but felt helpless to do anything about it.

DISSOCIATION AND SWITCHING

The internal system of an individual with DID is different for each person, yet very much the same. Switching can be a way of avoiding stress that seems overwhelming. In fact, dissociation in any form is a type of avoidance. (See Figure 9.1.)

The habitual use of dissociation or switching as a defense is based not only on perceived threats, but also on an individual's perceived ability to cope. Consequently, as your stress level rises, due to present circumstances or triggers related to past trauma, the key issue becomes whether you believe that you have resources available that will allow you to cope. If, at some level, you do not believe you have adequate resources, or if you are triggered at a physiological level, you may begin to switch internal states. (See Figure 9.2.)

The purpose of the avoidance related to dissociation is typically self-protection. One person may believe that he will lose control, or even die, if he allows himself to truly feel. So, when feelings begin to emerge, he dissociates. Another person's stress level rises and she

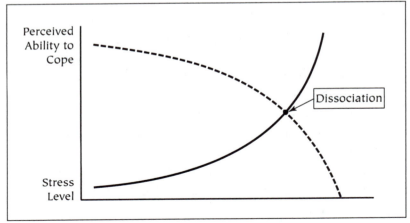

Figure 9.1 Haddock's Psychosocial Model of Dissociation

- Body becomes still or stiff.
- Person is slow to respond to others.
- Things seem to move in slow motion or fast-forward.
- Emotions become flat, numb; no feelings.
- Not feeling expected pain.
- Out of touch with surroundings.
- Drifts off, goes away, spaces out (gets spacey), blanks out, loses track of what's happening.
- Stares off into space, blank stare.
- Downward stare.
- Eyes dart anxiously from side to side or roll upward.
- Eyes blink rapidly or flutter.
- Faraway or dazed look.
- Tunes out.
- Not involved in present.
- Feels like an observer of the present situation, rather than a participant.

Figure 9.2 Possible Indications of Dissociation, *continued overleaf*

finds herself needing to set some limits, but does not know how. Dissociation is a way to temporarily escape the overwhelming feeling, thoughts of project deadlines, crying babies, or whatever the particular triggers might be.

There is a physiological component associated with dissociation that is trauma related and automatic, but there is a habitual aspect to the behavior as well. By consciously focusing on the dissociative behavior, you can begin to change it. The choice to avoid gets made at some level, often unconsciously. The problem is that if you choose to dissociate in an attempt to avoid, the "fix" is temporary and often creates further stress in the end. (See Figure 9.3.)

- Inattentive.
- Memory lapses.
- Fantasies, excessive daydreaming.
- Overactivity or withdrawal.
- Is on autopilot (automatism behavior); feels like a robot.
- Falls asleep.
- Disoriented.
- Misses conversation.
- Derealization (people or world do not seem real; feels like a stranger in a familiar place; does not recognize herself in the mirror; world seems like a dream, veiled).
- Feels as if one is watching things from outside one's body.
- Life split before and after (I'm a different person since the trauma).
- Twitches or grimaces.
- Clouds of alertness; foggy feeling (if you're suppressing traumas, you can't focus your thoughts; your mind goes blank).
- Unusual, inexplicable behavior (hits the ground when a car backfires; a dependable woman suddenly leaves the house for two days).
- Attempts to remain grounded in the present (strokes side of chair, taps, jiggles leg).
- Self-soothing (rocks back and forth).
- Things look or sound different: colors are faded or brighter, tunnel vision, wide-angle view, sounds are louder or more muffled than expected, things seem far away or unclear and fogged.

Reprinted with permission from *The Post-Traumatic Stress Disorder Sourcebook.* Copyright 2000.

Figure 9.2 Possible Indications of Dissociation, *continued*

Living in the present moment means accepting your experience, moment by moment, without judgment, which takes both practice and positive intention. The first step is simply to observe your behavior, without judgment. In the case of DID, as with everyone, that means observing the behaviors of which you are aware. With time, your sphere of awareness will gradually increase.

When people dissociate, they refer to it in various ways: spacing out, getting little, going away, and so on. They often feel as if they are floating, are outside of their bodies, or are lost in a fog. When that happens to you, take some time to answer the following questions:

1. What happened right before I started to dissociate?
2. What was I feeling, both physically and emotionally?
3. What is the last thing I remember?
4. I knew that I was dissociating because
   a. I started (tapping my foot, feeling dizzy, getting a headache, etc.);
   b. I stopped (talking, thinking clearly, making eye contact, etc.);
   c. I started to think (I'm going to die, people can't be trusted, I never do anything right, etc.).
5. What was I trying to avoid?
6. What else could I have done?

Initially, you may find you need help in answering some of these questions, but with practice, you will begin to identify the patterns associated with why and how your dissociation operates.

Figure 9.3 Practice Sheet for Staying in the Present Moment

There are some positive aspects to the behavior as well. Dissociation can be soothing in much the same way that some people find a glass of wine with dinner relaxing at the end of a stressful day. Switching to a younger part can be a great escape from the adult world of responsibilities and can illicit nurturing from the people closest to you. It can also allow parts to work on issues that are important to them and that may otherwise continue to go unnoticed. Dissociation can offer an individual the chance to say no to something when she feels unable to do so in any other way. It can also keep a person safe. Many dissociators have internal parts that keep others from committing suicide or harming themselves in other ways. Some parts exist solely to self-soothe. These aspects are good. Other coping strategies, however, will allow a person to stay present, which means more control, more empowerment, and less chaos (internally and externally) overall.

Increasing internal communication is the first step toward reaching that goal. DID clients sometimes express frustration because parts will not just disappear. Understand that each part that is experienced internally is a part of you, a person with DID. The goal is not to make them disappear, but to create more awareness and cooperation within the system. Awareness will increase gradually over time. There are various ways to make this happen, and it is important to try different techniques to see if a particular one works best.

INTERNAL COMMUNICATION TECHNIQUES

Writing in a journal is one internal communication technique. People have different styles. One possibility is to buy a notebook and make sections for each internal part. Then, when insights come or one part has information to communicate, a person can write it down in that section of the notebook. A variation of this technique is to buy a notebook and allow different parts to write in it as they wish. Sometimes the writing will take the form of questions for other parts, sometimes it will just be a way of expressing thoughts and feelings. But if it can take the form of a dialogue with other parts, it can become a very useful way of getting to know the whole self more fully. Increasing awareness also helps to decrease the internal barriers that lead to dissociation and switching.

Mapping the system can be another useful technique. Many therapists ask clients to map in the early stages of therapy as a way for both to gain a better understanding of how the system operates. An interesting aspect of this process is that maps tend to change over time; this serves as a nice representation of the changes that are occurring internally throughout the therapy process. (See Figure 9.4.)

Not all systems, however, are conducive to mapping; they are extremely fluid, and parts are not as distinct as in other systems. It is important for individuals to decide if mapping, or any other technique, is helpful for them. Doing exercises such as these solely to please the therapist may create more internal disruption.

It is also helpful for clients to take internal roll calls whenever needed. Usually, roll calls are met with resistance initially, in part because they challenge the purpose of the dissociation and can be experienced as a threat to the system. Most people, however, find this technique helpful with managing ambivalent feelings and with decision making. It also helps to identify where inner feelings or impulses are originating. A typical scenario is for a client to express a feeling, say, fear. The therapist might then ask why the client is feeling afraid. Often, the response is something akin to "I don't know." That may be because the fear is originating with another part; if so, many options are available at this point.

Sometimes a therapist will make contracts with individual parts. In this situation, the contract might be for one part to work on the feeling of fear for a portion of each session for the next month. It is

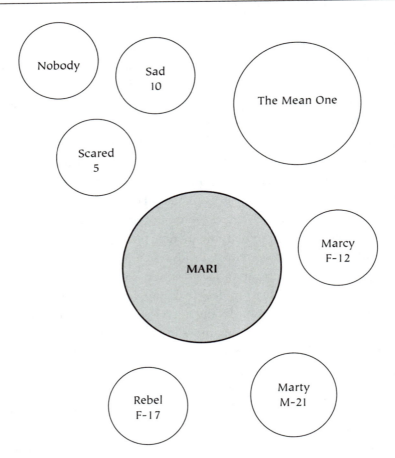

In session, Mari was asked to place herself in the middle and then allow others to put themselves where they felt they belonged. Sometimes alters will place themselves on the map, and sometimes they will ask someone else to do it, especially if they are younger. You can see from the map that some parts feel closer to each other than others do or they operate in similar ways. Some have put their age and gender. A therapist might also ask Mari to draw arrows that show which alters communicate with each other and whether the communication is two-way.

Figure 9.4 An Example of Mapping

important to think of the contract as two-way, between the individual part and the therapist, and three-way, among the individual part, the entire system, and the therapist. Because the true nature of a contract is an agreement between two or more people, with each offering something, the therapist needs to be willing to be an active participant as well. So, if this part is willing to work on fear, the therapist might agree to be more available by telephone during that time, and that becomes the contract between the two. For the entire system to be involved, it is important to get an agreement from other parts so that they will not interfere with this work. If this is difficult for some parts, they may need to join in the contract in a more formal way.

Another option at this point is to assign homework to a specific part. Again, if the issue is fear, the homework could be to list every major fear that part has, her specific thoughts about each of those fears, and what she would like to believe instead. (See Figure 9.5.)

The therapist might also instruct the client to check in with other parts who are older or less afraid so that they can be of help. This way, the individual alter is able to work through things, yet the overall goal of increasing internal communication is still being met. The therapist may also give the following instructions: "If there are specific things that keep you grounded (as opposed to dissociated) in the present, make a list and put it on a self-care card. Your list might include such things as cooking, doing laundry, or playing with the dog. That list sounds pretty mundane, doesn't it? Yet it is the ordinary things of life that keep us grounded in the present. Make a card of your own that includes your name, age, the current year, and at least five things that will help keep you grounded."

At times such as these, a therapist might suggest a roll call, asking the client to "go inside" and see which parts are present, what they are feeling, and whether they need anything. A roll call almost always helps the client identify the source of the feeling. Individuals can practice this technique whenever they feel disconnected from

Irrational Thoughts	Rational Thoughts
Fear 1: I am afraid that I will die if Mari (host) gets better.	
I will die if Mari gets better.	If Mari gets better, we will be more co-conscious, and that will be better for all of us.
Nobody cares about me.	We are all parts of one person. We're in this together.
Fear 2: I am afraid bad people are trying to hurt me.	
People from my past know where I live now, and they are looking for me.	I am an adult. The abusers from my past have no reason to be looking for me now.
The bad people know everything about me.	Abusers lie to children so that they won't talk about the abuse. Knowing everything about me is a lie. It is impossible.
I can't protect myself if something bad happens.	I am an adult, and I have more power now. I can make good decisions about how to keep myself safe. I have locks on my doors and windows. I have emergency phone numbers programmed into my telephones.

Figure 9.5 Homework: Marcy's Fears

or confused by their feelings. They can also use it when they are experiencing a lot of ambivalence with a decision they need to make, however small. If you experience dissociation and would like to implement this technique, start by making yourself as comfortable as possible. If it feels safe, close your eyes and take two or three deep breaths. Then, one by one, check in to see which parts are present. Depending on how your system works, you may see parts, hear them, or simply sense their presence. How the process occurs does not really matter, as long as containment skills have been practiced in therapy and internal safety can be established. The purpose of the exercise is to slow yourself down, increase internal awareness, and learn how to make conscious decisions. It is very important to listen to internal parts with a nonjudgmental attitude so that they will feel free to continue to speak. With DID, all parts are important aspects of the Self and exist for a reason, even if it is hard to understand or accept that concept early in treatment.

A variation of the roll call is to visualize a meeting room of some kind. Some people use a conference room and imagine each part taking a seat at the conference table. An internal microphone or spotlight can be used as a way of focusing attention on each part, allowing them all to contribute to the meeting.[1] Some people describe having an elaborate internal system with each part having personal space inside. If internal parts live in a house and operate like a family, the meeting place might be in the family room or around the kitchen table. Instead of a spotlight, an internal secretary can be appointed to take roll. Using whatever technique is most helpful is what counts. Most important, checking in at least once a day and rotating leadership at the meetings will increase cooperative communication among parts.

BASIC SAFETY PLAN

The most successful safety plans are those tailored to a client's specific needs. Better yet, both the client and therapist develop them. People who dissociate tend to experience a lot of personal chaos in the early stages of therapy, but they have not developed the degree of trust necessary to be able to communicate needs clearly. Thus, the first step is to create a safe place, both inside and out. Then the task is to develop a basic safety plan that can be changed as the therapeutic relationship grows and as more information is gleaned.

A basic safety plan includes how to deal with emergencies. It is also a good idea to define *emergency* from the beginning. Therapists have different styles as well as differing beliefs about what is appropriate for the clients with whom they work. Some therapists use voice mail or pager systems, some use answering services, and others allow clients to call a home number if this does not become intrusive. Any of these options is workable, but it is important for clients to begin to develop a support network immediately. If you rely solely on the therapist to meet all your needs, you become disappointed and may feel resentful when you find that he cannot.

The first step, then, is to determine what the initial safety plan will cover. The therapist's role is to decide his after-hours availability. Then, together, you and your therapist can decide what words such as *crisis* or *emergency*, will mean. It can be helpful to have a short brainstorming session in which you can talk about what types of issues might come up for you when you are away from your therapist's office. Issues might include self-injurious behaviors, suicidal gestures, flashbacks, a younger part emerging in the middle of the night, and getting lost on the way home from a therapy session.

After making the list, both you and your therapist can brainstorm again about all the possible people who could offer support during a crisis. This list can include the therapist, friends, family, a pastor, and members from a support group. A crisis line can also be a good resource if the therapist is familiar with one that is good and if someone inside is able to take charge and communicate effectively. If not, crisis lines can sometimes create more problems because the person on the other end of the line may not fully understand the reason for the call. If a younger part calls and is talking about wanting to die and the counselor on the other end does not understand that you have DID and that wanting to die may not actually be a suicide threat, he may have no other choice than to call the police. It could be helpful to discuss crisis lines with your therapist rather than randomly calling one listed in the telephone book. It could also be helpful to brainstorm again about some basic self-soothing behaviors you can use if you find yourself in a crisis situation. The basic plan has three components:

1. Name the behavior.
2. List five to ten self-soothing behaviors that can be used to manage emotions.
3. List people to call, if needed.

Figure 9.6 is a typical safety plan.

Figure 9.7 provides space to try a safety plan of your own. Be as specific as possible and remember to name the behavior, list some self-soothing activities, and list people you can call if needed.

---

1. If I feel suicidal and don't believe I can control my impulses, I will begin to step back and slow myself down by

    a. taking a warm bath and listening to soothing music;
    b. calling a friend;
    c. making some popcorn and watching my favorite movie;
    d. taking a roll call and seeing if a particular part is upset—if so, I will do something soothing for that part;
    e. going to bed early and snuggling up with my favorite stuffed animal.

2. If, after trying these things, I still need help, I will call

    a. my best friend, Carla, at (phone number);
    b. my friend, John, from my depression group at (phone number);
    c. my therapist, at (phone number)

Figure 9.6 Sample Safety Plan

(List behavior.)

(List at least five self-soothing activities for each part, remembering that the system, as a whole, can share activities.)

(List three to five people to call.)

Figure 9.7 My Basic Safety Plan

If you have worked on a safety plan on your own, share it with your therapist and key support people. The more these issues are discussed, the safer you will feel. Sandra Hocking gives an example of a detailed contract for survival, reproduced in Figure 9.8, in her book *Living with Your Selves.*

Self-Care Cards

The safety plan should be carried at all times. A small spiral book of note cards that can be easily slipped into a purse or backpack can be the beginning of your self-care kit. On the first cards, write down the basic safety plan modeled after Figure 9.7. Also include a card that can serve as a reminder of your current age and the current year, such as the one illustrated in Figure 9.9.

To cover the period of _____ to _____

I/We _____

agree not to knowingly or intentionally cause serious or fatal bodily harm or injury, including those actions which could result therein (i.e., overdose, reckless driving, etc.) to this physical, mental, emotional or spiritual body. I/We will not knowingly kill, physically, mentally, emotionally or spiritually, ourselves or any other person or personality.

As protectors, we the undersigned, to the best of our ability, agree to intervene on behalf of our other persons or personalities who may be unable or unwilling to do so, by calling and actually reaching and connecting with the support members listed on this form.

When I call a support person, I will state that I am calling because of the contract and we will honestly address and discuss the emotions and events that led to crisis and the possible solutions and safety measures to be taken. We will continue to pursue all phone numbers, including repetitions, until the crisis is resolved.

In the event of breaking or attempting to break this contract, professional intervention may be contacted and requested.

Anyone who has reservations about signing this contract must voice them now or be bound by this contract for the duration of the contract period.

This contract is valid past the end date until a new contract has been negotiated or all support members of the previously agreed-upon contract have been contacted and agree that relinquishment of this contract is in the best interests of the contractee.

Signature of Host Personality:_____

Signatures of those who agree to intervene on behalf of the host and others in the system:

_____

_____

_____

Figure 9.8 Contract for Survival   *Continued overleaf*

I object to the signing of this contract. I will discuss my reasons here:

_____

_____

_____

_____

These are the persons/agencies I agree to call:

Name and Phone Number

_____

_____

_____

_____

I, the undersigned support person(s), agree to provide emotional or physical support to the contractee within the terms of this contract. I understand the contractee may contact me any time of the day or night.

_____

_____

_____

Reprinted with permission from *Living with Your Selves* by Sandra J. Hocking. Copyright 1992 Launch Press.

Figure 9.8 Contract for Survival, *continued*

Some other ideas for things to include on self-care cards are listed in Figure 9.10, a compilation of grounding techniques.

As therapy progresses, you will become more aware of how your own internal systems operate. This point is the time for making cards that address how to deal with specific issues, such as managing flashbacks. These cards will go a step beyond the basic safety plan and will be tailored to each person's individual needs and the

My name is Mari.
I am thirty-nine years old and the year is 2001.

Figure 9.9 Self-Care Card

way her specific system operates. An example of a self-care card for managing flashbacks is shown in Figure 9.11.

Of course, even the best-laid plans will fail at times, especially in the early stages of therapy. In the beginning stage of therapy, dissociation can often happen before you even realize it, flashbacks occur, and sometimes it is hard to even remember you have cards to look at, but do not despair! Therapy is a learning process. You will be able to learn something about yourself even when your self-care plan gets tossed aside. Dissociation has been a lifesaving defense. The goal is to learn to understand how it works in your life so that you can make conscious choices about how you want to respond to present triggers. In the future, with practice, you will begin to recognize the signs of dissociation and will be able to slow yourself down early enough to implement some of the suggestions on your cards. Make the cards inviting so that you will want to use them and so that they will appeal to younger parts as well. Individual parts might even want to make cards of their own. Use bright colors. Be

Use these techniques when you begin dissociating. The goal is to begin using them sooner and sooner so that you can eventually make use of them at the first hint of an emotion that might be difficult for you, such as anxiety. Be sure to add your own ideas to the list.

- Keep your eyes open and your feet on the ground.
- Hold a stuffed animal or other comforting object.
- Hold something that is cold or put a bag of frozen vegetables on your neck.
- Listen to calming music.
- Pray, very specifically, about what you need right now. It takes more concentration to be specific. The serenity prayer can be helpful too.
- In a public place, tune in to another voice, provided it is either neutral or calming
- If alone, consider calling a friend.
- Remind yourself of the difference between then and now by saying the date out loud, naming where you are, and saying your age. It is good to have calendars and pictures of yourself as an adult throughout the house.
- Create a safe place inside where you can image when feeling dissociated.
- Breathe mindfully, focusing on each inhalation and each exhalation. Breathe with your eyes open.
- Do something that involves each of your senses, such as reading, watching television, touching a worry stone, smelling a flower, or eating sunflower seeds.
- Choose a grounding phrase that you can say to yourself, such as "I'm an adult now and I'm safe."
- Listen to a tape of your therapist's voice.
- Do a behavior chain, or something similar, that will help you to understand what triggered you and how you might be able to handle it differently in the future.
- Carry a small medicine bag with objects that are meaningful to you.
- Go for a walk.

Figure 9.10 Sample Grounding Techniques

- Do something with your hands, such as drawing, gardening, a cross-word puzzle, writing in a journal, or painting.

- Take a shower.

- Don't forget younger parts. Read to them or play a cassette of lullabies or a story read by your therapist. Snuggle up in bed and hold a stuffed animal and watch cartoons.

- Keep adding to the list.

- Be compassionate toward yourself, open and without judgment. You deserve kindness!

Figure 9.10 Sample Grounding Techniques, *continued*

artistic. Include inspiring quotes that motivate you and lift your spirits. Recognize that by being proactive, you are already experiencing success!

Now let's try a card for managing suicidal thoughts. (See Figure 9.12.)

1. Roll call. If someone inside is upset, I will do something to soothe that part. (One suggestion is to make a self-soothing card for each part so that it is there when you need it. In the midst of crisis or overwhelming feelings it can be difficult to think clearly.)

2. I will identify the thoughts that are making me want to hurt myself. (Suicidal thoughts might represent angry thoughts toward yourself or negative messages from long ago. They might also be about internal conflicts among ego states, or they may be misbeliefs that can be redirected with the help of others. Sometimes internal parts truly believe they would be better off dead and that their death will help the host or some other part. This thinking is logical in the midst of terrifying abuse, although illogical now. It is equally important to have a "We're in this together" attitude if you want to overcome past conditioning or ineffective coping methods.)

---

1. Ask other parts inside for help.
2. Breathe deeply.
3. Refer to card on staying grounded in the present.
4. Create safety inside for younger parts by
   - reading a bedtime story and letting an internal helper tuck them safely away inside;
   - expressing gratitude for all the hard work they did for you in the past and reassuring them about their safety in the present;
   - reminding them that older parts can handle the situation now.

Figure 9.11 Flashbacks

3. I will make a list of feelings I am having and remind my-self that feelings will not kill me.
4. I will call someone just to talk or, if possible, get together with someone. (Be specific and include the phone numbers of several people right on the card.)

Now, make a list of situations or behaviors for which you might need a card on hand to coach you. Then make two or three cards to share with your therapist. Continue to make new cards as issues arise. Here are a few examples of situations you might put on a card. Pick two or three from the list or choose one of your own for practice.

1. Being assertive with my boss when he asks me to work late.
2. Telling my mother that I do not want to talk right now.
3. Dealing with younger parts that want to come out in public.
4. Turning the feeling thermometer down when I start to feel overwhelmed.
5. Turning the television channel to safety.
6. Not drinking alcohol.
7. Handling paralyzing fear in the middle of the night.

Managing suicidal thoughts

_____

_____

_____

_____

_____

_____

_____

_____

Figure 9.12 Suicidal Thoughts

8. Becoming excessively startled in the middle of the day.
9. Identifying behaviors to use in place of bingeing.
10. Establishing daily goals for health and well-being.

ACCEPTING INTERNAL PARTS

It is important to focus on roll calls, how to soothe parts, and internal communication, because respecting and nurturing parts is one of the keys to getting healthier. If you have DID, you can probably identify with the concept of "getting rid of" parts. There are variations on the theme, but the concept centers on wanting to be "normal" and undoing what has happened in the past. Being healthier is a great goal, but you need to ask yourself what normal means to you. If it means living the shared human experience, normal means having good and bad feelings and good and bad times. It might also mean living with things you do not particularly like and learning how to accept and manage those situations. When M. Scott Peck opened his book *The Road Less Traveled* with the words "Life is difficult," it surprised me initially. "Come on," I said, "People want to hear good things. We want to find out how to overcome whatever it is in life that we do not like. Don't tell me that life is difficult." Yet it is.

In Buddhist teaching, the first noble truth states that life is suffering. In Christian teaching, Jesus said not to be surprised when troubles come our way. In fact, all great spiritual teachers start by recognizing the situation as it is; only then can something be done about it. If your desire is to be a full participant in the human race, know that it is only by accepting the reality of your life that you will be able to do so. Begin by accepting that life has dealt you a difficult hand. You have advanced to a certain seat in the tournament. Now you have reached the round of play where increasing awareness of who you are is what is going to keep you in the game.

If you are still undecided about whether to stay in the game, practice accepting yourself wherever you are. You do not have to make a decision right now about where you want to be five years from now; you only have to agree to work on the issues that are presenting themselves today. If you do that with integrity, you will know when it is time to make further decisions about the direction of your life.

Working with internal parts starts with awareness, which leads to understanding and, finally, acceptance. Therapists do not help clients to get rid of any part of themselves. Even if they tried to, it would not work. Remember the mapping exercise? Just continue to build on that. Think of mapping as the foundation on which you are going to build and then work at purposeful or conscious communication. Use the various communication techniques discussed in this chapter on a regular basis. Move into an even deeper level of communication. Such communication is like the difference between having a casual relationship with someone and then moving into a deeper friendship.

Two components in relationships are especially pertinent to the topic of self-help and coping: respect and nurturing. Hence, the reason for not ignoring or getting rid of parts is that the role of a part can change over time, which is very different from ceasing to exist. Integration itself is about change, not the extinction of parts.

Respect has to do with appreciation for the work that was done to ensure your survival. It might include actually naming things each part has done. "Thank you, Betsy, for being present when Tim abused me and I wasn't able to stay present. You made it possible for me to stay alive." Eventually, you will be able to see that Betsy is not a separate person but is very much a part of you. Or, as an adult, you might have difficulty tolerating feelings. "Thanks, Mary, for setting limits with my father when I am afraid to do so." Someday you will find that you will not have to switch to set limits, because you and Mary will be able to operate as one.

The other component is nurturing. If increased internal awareness never occurs, other parts can begin to grow weary of playing their roles, but if you offer time off and appreciation for work done, you can begin to function much like an internal family. It can be extremely helpful to read a bedtime story to a child part, to allow a teenage part to play loud music while you are cleaning house, or to let one part read trashy novels even though you prefer Jane Austen. The end result of an affirming attitude is less internal chaos and negative competition, which results in better functioning overall.

Some people find it helpful to collect objects that are especially soothing or representational of internal parts. You might have a special area in your house where you keep these things, a kind of time-out room. You might even carry things such as a stuffed animal for a younger part, a religious symbol, a favorite quote, a picture of someone you love, or a healing stone with you in your purse or car. You might adopt a pet to keep you company at home. Different parts might even make artistic creations that help with self-soothing. You can fill your home with these objects to remind yourself that you are safe. These things not only soothe; they also serve as constant reminders that you are connected to this world. It can also be helpful to carry transitional objects (remember Linus and his blanket?) that help you feel connected to your therapist. Objects such as cards, a small trinket, a stuffed animal, rocks, or shells may help you stay connected to your therapist when you are away from the office.

> I have incorporated self-soothing, centering techniques as well as imagery into my treatment. When I am on vacation, I also offer my clients transitional objects to keep while I am gone. For some, journalizing and drawing have been helpful. I need to continually assess where my clients are and, at different stages of recovery, some techniques are more beneficial than others.
> (Judith, therapist, Canada)

You might also want to include things that remind you of other people who love you. Many people have photo albums filled with pictures of people who love them and places that feel safe. These types of things will help you remember the "heart connection" you have with others if it becomes difficult to feel a connection with your inner self.

ORGANIZING INFORMATION
FOR FAMILY AND FRIENDS

In the early stages of therapy, it can feel lonely and overwhelming to be dealing with difficult issues and an internal system that others are not even aware exists. Some clients say they want to feel connected to people yet fear rejection if anyone gets too close. The "getting too close" is usually a reference to having DID. Many people carry a sense of shame about having this diagnosis and believe people will think of them as odd or sick if the reality of their experience is shared. Sadly, this reaction can happen, but not in every case. You need to think very carefully about whom you want to share your diagnosis with and why. This topic is an excellent one to explore in therapy. It is important to move slowly and be clear about your own goals rather than sharing information with others that you might later regret. Yet sharing information with those who are closest to you, and known to be safe, is vital if you want to reduce the stress associated with hiding your dissociation. Sharing is also a way of getting some of the support you need. It is a form of healthy connecting. People with whom you might consider sharing your diagnosis are a loving partner, close friend, roommate, family member, or health care provider. The person needs to be someone you trust and with whom you truly want to be more connected. An example of how to organize the information that you want to share is given in Figure 9.13.

IMAGERY FOR MANAGING FEELINGS

Think of feelings as being neutral. They are simply providing you with information about your experience. You are not your feelings. You are merely experiencing something called anxiety, sadness, and so on. One helpful technique for managing emotions is to image them. You might imagine overwhelming emotion as being like a wave. If you simply sit and allow the wave to wash over you, you will be safe and the emotion will pass. Only when you try to fight the wave of emotion will you begin to feel as though you might be pulled under.

Dear _____ (name of person),

Because you know that I am dissociative, I'd like to be able to share some information with you about my DID so that you will know me better. Please don't share the information with anyone else, but if you want to talk about it with me, I'm open to that. I trust you and care about you, which is why I'm choosing to share this information about myself with you. Thanks for being a part of my life!

My internal system:

Alter's name, age, brief description, and how he or she might be recognized.

    Alter #1: _____

    Alter #2: _____

(Continue to list parts that you know or parts that are likely to interact with this person. Check inside to see who wants to be included.)

Things I need from you if possible:

If you think I've switched, just ask.

If I seem younger, ask if you can sit by me. Offer me my favorite stuffed animal if it seems to help.

Be real. Don't take responsibility for my feelings. Just be present.

Ask for an adult to come out if you need to do so.

Figure 9.13 Template for Sharing

Or, you might give the emotion a particular shape and color, provided you are aware of any past shapes and colors that could be triggering for you. Notice where you feel it in your body. Then imagine a white light (or whatever color seems most healing or comforting to you) entering your body through the top of your head and traveling completely through your body until it reaches the very tips of your

---

Vital information:

My therapist's name is: _____ (name of therapist).

Her phone number is: _____ (therapist's phone number). You can call her if there is an emergency.

My medications are (list medications; be sure to include dosages):

Things I want you to know about me:

1. I love the theater.

2. I don't want to switch when I'm with you, although I know it's a possibility.

3.

4.

Things I wish for our relationship:

1. I want our friendship to grow on an adult-to-adult basis.

2. I want to do something fun with you once or twice a month.

3.

4.

Figure 9.13 Template for Sharing, *continued*

toes. As the healing light travels through your body, allow it to interact with the overwhelming emotions. Just notice whatever happens. *Caution:* Do not use this exercise if you tend to be triggered by shapes or colors.

You might also image your emotions as a wise teacher who has come to pay you a visit. What does the teacher look like? Allow the wise teacher to speak to you without any reservation or judgment on your part.

You could pretend that the emotion is an animal: an angry lion, a sad little puppy, an anxious monkey. In your mind, reach out to the animal and try to understand it better. You might even want to draw a picture that illustrates the way the animal is presenting itself to you.

Maybe there is a way of imaging your emotions that fits your particular personality or style. Take out a piece of paper and think of an emotion you would like to be more aware of or one with which you would like to feel more comfortable. Use crayons to image the emotion. Title your drawing. Now decide how you want to work with the image the next time it appears: "The next time I feel anxious . . ."

Finally, consider doing a collage about the feeling or issue with which you are dealing. Be sure to invite all parts to get involved. Then share the collage with your therapist.

A HEALTHY LIFESTYLE
AS A STRATEGY FOR COPING

Taking the best care of yourself you possibly can may be the most practical coping strategy there is. Eating properly, getting enough sleep, and including time for relaxation every day is a must. Exercising at least three times a week will help regulate your mood and will increase your overall level of well-being. Exercise is a great energy booster. Do what you can to eliminate negative habits. Decrease or totally eliminate caffeine from your diet, recognizing that caffeine can increase your anxiety level, cause headaches, and disrupt your sleep. If you smoke, ask your doctor about ways to quit or contact the Hazelden Foundation in Center City, Minnesota, about resources for quitting (see appendix B). Consider taking a daily vitamin supplement and drinking plenty of water (eight glasses a day is recommended) to clear your body of toxins and replace the necessary minerals needed for good health. Work slowly on making these changes. It is too overwhelming to attempt to change your lifestyle completely, and this is usually easier to address later in therapy.

A healthy lifestyle will equip you to handle stress better when it does invade your life. Even small attempts at lifestyle change can help. You can start by setting small goals that you can practice one day at a time. Initially, such goals can increase stress because you are asking yourself to do something different. Most people can name at least one thing they do to relieve stress that is not very healthy. It is never easy to stop using that favorite coping technique. If you live on junk food, cigarettes, and caffeine, you will find that your body begins to flush toxins from its system when you start eating healthier foods. Physically, this process can feel like a crisis, but if you stay with it, you will find that response is truly short lived. In addition, the payoff is enormous. By practicing a healthier lifestyle, you actually begin to experience less emotional stress.

You might also want to consider adding a spiritual practice at least once a week and connecting with friends at least that often as well. Andrew Weil's *Eight Weeks to Optimum Health* gives such practical suggestions as having fresh flowers in your home and listening to inspirational music daily. He also suggests taking a news fast from time to time so that you are not constantly polluting your mind with negative thoughts. It can feel very empowering to recognize that you have the ability to set a mood of health and positive intention both within and throughout your environment.

SUMMARY

Self-help and coping techniques are an essential part of therapy for people who dissociate. Not only do these techniques help you to stay safe, but they also aid you in gaining mastery over difficult situations. With each positive step, you will feel more self-empowered.

You can begin by using the techniques discussed in this chapter, but feel free to adapt them in whatever way is most useful for you and then begin to add things you come up with on your own. The following list is an excellent beginning:

- Increase internal communication among parts by writing in a journal mapping your internal system, and taking roll calls or holding internal family meetings regularly.
- Develop a basic safety plan and put it in writing.
- Create note cards to use when feeling overwhelmed or in need of encouragement.
- Practice nurturing, respecting, and expressing gratitude to internal parts.
- Collect objects that are soothing and empowering and carry them with you.
- Let support people know what is helpful for you.
- Use imagery, meditation, or DBT skills for managing feelings.
- Use meditation books or other inspirational writings for encouragement and grounding.
- Exercise to improve mood and overall sense of well-being.

Above all else, do everything in moderation. The goal is progress, not perfection!

Chapter Ten

Survival Tips for Significant Others (and Therapists Too)

Although this chapter is addressed specifically to the significant people in the lives of those with DID—friends, family members, and therapists—it is also offered as a means of opening communication among the person experiencing dissociation and the people with whom they are in relationships.

Knowing someone with DID can be rewarding, interesting, challenging, and at times downright frustrating. Friends comment that Lori's mood swings are confusing. They are never quite sure what to expect when they spend time with her.

Marsha's partner says that one of the reasons their relationship is so interesting is because Marsha is multidimensional. There is never a dull moment. He admits that it can be a little disconcerting to walk into the house only to be greeted by a child in a thirty-year-old body. Yet he is quick to add, "She is the person I married, and we will learn to work through it together."

John's therapist admits that he never planned to treat DID patients, but over the course of his practice he has treated several. "DID patients can be challenging, to say the least, but I think I have learned more about myself from my DID patients than from anyone else," he says. "I have learned the importance of being fully present with a patient, and it has taught me to be more fully present with myself."

BASIC COMMUNICATION

A relationship with someone with DID is like any other relationship: you have to define your parameters. If it is a close relationship with a friend or family member, you need to decide how to deal with the dissociative symptoms. In some relationships, the participants try to pretend that the DID does not exist. Usually, that simply serves to increase the stress. It is akin to the pink elephant in the living room; everybody knows that it is there but nobody wants to say anything. Some people choose to accept the dissociation to the point that interaction with alters is a normal part of the relationship. In these relationships, the person with the DID might choose to switch in front of the other person and the other person will interact with whatever part is out. In other relationships, the DID is acknowledged, but the nondissociator does not normally communicate with parts and may not even know, at times, that they are present. He may observe switching, but he addresses the host and does not get overly involved with individual parts. Whether you interact with these parts is a decision that needs to be made between you and your friend or family member. There is nothing inherently wrong with communication with parts, but it is important that you not assume a caretaker role with the dissociator in your life. When a friend or partner does so, he runs the risk of becoming more like a therapist or parent. When that happens, the relationship becomes unbalanced and resentments can easily build. Whatever your relationship, it needs to be built on trust, clarity, and mutual respect within the context of adult communication.

Anyone who is involved in a relationship with someone with DID will experience a gamut of emotions. It is important to remember that two separate people are involved. The same boundaries apply to DID as to any other relationship, but it is not possible to be in a relationship with someone with DID and not be affected. The internal conflicts experienced by someone who dissociates will be noticeable to the people closest to her even if no one is able to name what is happening. The "not naming" might have to do with not wanting to deal with reality, but more often it is probably about not understanding what is happening. When internal conflicts occur for someone with DID, many things can happen. The experience can be as minor as a disagreement among parts (a sort of internal civil war that causes some confusion or mood changes) or it can become extremely chaotic, both inside and out. At such times, the person who is dissociating may be hearing so many voices inside her head that it becomes difficult to concentrate. She may experience several emotions at the same time as internal parts vie to be heard and take control. You might notice rapid switching at these times as well as behavior that is confusing or seemingly unrelated to the outward experience. At its most extreme, internal conflicts can lead to impulsive acting out or self-harm (drinking, rage, cutting, bingeing, and purging). People describe this internal experience in different ways, but all agree that it is a difficult and often frightening place to be. Some people talk about wanting to get "little" so that someone will comfort them. Others talk about wanting to isolate so that no one will see what they are going through. Almost without exception there is a pervasive sense of shame, not only about being DID but also about even being alive. People with DID need to be encouraged to reach out to friends, family, or other support people whom they know to be safe when they are struggling internally, yet shame often keeps them from doing so. For many, there is a fear that sharing that deep hurt and internal struggle will only serve to leave them vulnerable to rejection from the people they care about the most.

- My husband deserves better. He shouldn't have to live like this.
- My father does not want to deal with it. He does not even believe I have DID.
- If anybody knew about it my career would be ruined.
- Nobody understands how much energy it takes for me to make it through every day, but who can I tell? Nobody wants to be friends with someone who has so many problems.

If you have a person with DID in your life, learn whatever you can about the disorder from reputable sources such as those listed in appendix B. Then tell your friend or family member you are willing to be available to hear the truth of whatever it is he is going through. If you are not sure you can do that, decide what you can do and communicate it honestly. This process is an example of appropriate boundary setting. People with DID are survivors, and they are very sensitive to dishonesty in relationships. Being willing to learn about the disorder and being genuine as you relate to the other person are the most important things you can offer.

BOUNDARY ISSUES

Certain boundary issues immediately present themselves when you begin a relationship with someone who has DID. In therapy, the first of those issues is frequency of telephone calls. From time to time, people with DID will find themselves experiencing feelings with which they do not feel prepared to deal. Sometimes they may experience extreme fear related to flashbacks. Other times they might feel what could be considered normal human emotions, even though they are experienced as overwhelming and unmanageable to the person who has the feelings. Strong emotions can trigger feelings of powerlessness and abandonment that the average person simply cannot understand. No therapist wants clients to have to experience that kind of distress. Yet responding to every call only helps increase the client's feelings of dependency and powerlessness. The key is to create clear boundaries initially that can be reworked as needed.

Clients will need to know if, at a certain time each night, the therapist will be unavailable, but they also need to know that other options exist, such as voice mail or an answering service. Often, being able to leave a message on the therapist's voice mail and knowing that it will be heard is enough. Yet it can also be helpful for clients to know that at any time they can say, "I am not just checking in right now. I really need you to call me." Then, if possible, the therapist can call and spend ten to fifteen minutes working on containment of the emotions. If the therapist is not immediately available and the appropriate stabilization work has been done, the client knows that a plan is already in place for times like these. The most important aspect is that a plan is developed conjointly between therapist and client, based on the client's ability to manage emotions and the stage of therapy. This plan is then coupled with enough flexibility on the part of the therapist to operate outside the box when needed.

This way of dealing with telephone calls is not the only way. Some therapists use answering services exclusively, others share on-call responsibilities with a group of therapists, and others make a home number available. What is important is being clear about what is acceptable and what kind of help can reasonably be provided over the phone.

What happens, however, if you have a friend who has DID and you do not have an answering service to take the calls? Honesty is indeed the best policy. Talk with your friend about when it is acceptable or not acceptable to call. If she calls and you are busy, politely say so. Decide together what the limitations of your friendship will be. Here are two examples of appropriate boundaries that a friend might set:

- I will be glad to chat for thirty minutes now and then if you are having problems, but please do not call after 7:00 in the evening on weeknights because that is usually when I spend time with my family.
- If you are feeling afraid or lonely, give me a call. If it is possible, you can come over and watch television or something even if I am busy doing other things. Maybe being around other people will help you feel safer.

Honest adult communication and negotiation is what is needed so that significant others do not take on the role of therapist. Once that happens, the friendship is likely to become strained.

Switching is another boundary issue in these types of relationships. If you live with someone who has DID, does it mean you have to be constantly alert to which part is out? The answer is no. The responsibility really lies with the person experiencing the dissociation. Some people choose to always address a friend with DID by the host's name regardless of who is presenting. Others address the various ego states by name if they are asked to do so. It simply is not reasonable to expect to live with someone who has DID and not have him or her switch; this is who she is. It is reasonable, however, to talk about how you might interact with other parts. If a child part will feel safer if you cuddle her and both you and your partner are comfortable with that, it might be a good idea. Yet it is also important for the person who dissociates to have space of her own in the house that can be considered a safe place. That way, if switching feels as if it might be unduly interfering with others in the family, the dissociative person can take a time out in her own safe place, with or without you. Ideally, she will be able to communicate that she is taking a time out.

Another good strategy is to build safety into the various rooms of the house. You can help your roommate or family member choose calming things, such as a stack of coloring books or crossword puz-

zles, to keep in the family room. Then, if your friend or loved one begins to feel afraid or agitated inside while the family is talking or watching television, she can choose a calming activity to do as a way of
soothing herself. Or, she might have a certain radio station she listens
to while working in the kitchen. If a part of her self wants to withdraw
when feeling angry, she could wear headphones and listen to alternative rock while another part is doing something else. Making such al-
lowances for someone helps her manage feelings in a safe way that still
allows the rest of the family to function somewhat normally. It is also a
respectful way of helping everyone in the house get their needs met.

Inherent in either of these situations, however, can be the spoken
or unspoken demand by your friend or loved one to be taken care of.
This demand could be a form of manipulation, or it could be a genuine
belief she has in her own inability to deal with whatever situation is
presenting itself. Taking care of another adult is generally not advisable
because it sends the message that she really is not able to deal effectively with life, and it is disempowering. It is far better to walk the person through whatever she is facing, being clear about what you will and
will not do, and asking her to be clear about what she needs so that
you can respond honestly. We are all dependent on each other to some
degree or another. The way to make that work is by making clear requests and by responding clearly to requests that are made. What happens, though, when the formula fails? Continually discuss this
possibility with the dissociator in your life and work together to develop creative solutions. Here are some possibilities to get you started:

- Decide on a code word that means "Remember your safe
  place." (The safe place can be literal or a place in the mind.
  Most people who dissociate differentiate between "inside"
  and "outside."
- I need for (host's name) to come close enough so that I can
  communicate with her.

- It seems like you are feeling (insert name of feeling), but I cannot help you until an adult part can let me know what's needed. Please go inside and ask for an adult part to come out.
- I do not know what you need right now. Let's sit together on the couch and watch television until you are feeling better and able to talk.

One communication issue that can be especially challenging is dealing with passive-aggressive communication. Passive-aggressive communication includes an element of unexpressed anger that is communicated indirectly. (See Table 10.1.)

Everyone has probably been passive-aggressive at some point. It certainly is not unique to DID. If you are on the receiving end of passive-aggressive communication, your feelings may range from confusion to anger. It is the indirectness of the communication that is so difficult to handle. Boundaries can be difficult to maintain in a passive-aggressive relationship because it can be easy to get pulled into a power struggle. Yet when boundaries are difficult to maintain, that is probably when they are most important. Whether your role is that of therapist or friend, you need to let the dissociative person know that you can only respond directly to what is being presented directly. Do not become the caretaker, expending energy on guessing what the other person needs. The following examples illustrate passive-aggressive behavior on the parts of Peter and Donna. Notice how you might feel if you were on the receiving end of this form of communication.

Peter wanted to go to a ball game with some friends. He listened to them talking about their plans, but instead of asking if he could join them, he became sullen and withdrawn. Cole noticed and asked him if something was wrong, without even

Table 10.1 Passive Versus Assertive Communication Styles

Passive	Assertive
Indirect and emotionally dishonest.	Emotionally honest and direct in a way that is respectful of the other person.
Denies ability or right to make own choices.	Accepts responsibility for making own choices.
Poor eye contact, soft voice, almost childlike in style of communication.	Appropriate eye contact, relaxed, adult-to-adult style of communication.
A belief that she cannot get or do not deserve what she wants, so she communicates indirectly, which often ends up reinforcing the belief.	A belief that all people are worthwhile and entitled to their opinions. Communicates openly and with a win–win attitude.
Ends up feeling disappointed and powerless. Often feels angry toward the other person because personal goals have not been reached.	Often feels confident and pleased about end results because both parties are able to feel that part or all of their personal goals have been reached.

realizing that Peter might have been feeling left out. Although Peter looked angry, his voice sounded flat and without emotion when he answered by saying, "Oh, sorry. Everything is fine." He then did his best to avoid Cole for the next few days. Cole knew something was wrong, but he had no idea what it was. He mentioned the behavior to Peter once again, but when he was met with a curt denial of any negative feelings, Cole realized that the issue was really Peter's to deal with. He continued to interact with Peter as normally as possible, but he didn't attempt to pressure him any further about his behavior.

Donna was looking forward to a night out with some friends. She wanted her husband, Joe, to stay home with the kids, which he would have gladly done if only he had known about Donna's plans. As it turned out, both of them had made plans with friends for the same night. With a little problem solving the situation could have been handled, but Donna was so angry about the mix-up that she simply canceled her own plans and told Joe that she would be willing to stay home. It was not a big deal, she told him. She seemed so sincere that he believed her, but two days later as Joe was getting ready to go out, Donna flew into a rage about how unfair he was being to her by making her stay home. Joe calmly reminded her of the chain of events leading to her decision to stay at home and said he would be happy to talk about it the next day. Then he mentally left the conflict at home and enjoyed the evening with his friends.

Another difficult issue is when someone in your life creates a crisis. Creating a crisis can be conscious or unconscious. It is a way of turning up the heat so that someone will respond. Picture a two-year-old playing in the kitchen while his mother is fixing dinner. He notices that no one is paying attention to him, so he starts tugging at her leg. She continues to chop carrots. The child starts to feel anxious because she is still not paying attention to him. Now he is slapping her leg and whimpering. If the mother stops for a minute and talks to him or picks him up, things will probably be okay. If not, a full-blown temper tantrum may ensue. That is a two-year-old's way of saying, "I need you, and I feel mad and scared when you do not respond."

Something similar happens at times for the person with DID. He may indeed feel two years old himself. Or, he might feel older, but deficient in the skills needed to get his needs met. Like a two-year-old, he begins to act out his fears and rage in an effort to get you to respond. That effort might present itself as verbal threats, infliction of self-harm, or even suicidal gestures. Let's be honest; it is hard not to respond if you believe someone is in danger. The challenge is to respond appropriately. Some ways you could respond while keeping your own boundaries intact include the following:

- Reminding her of her safe place, both inside and outside, if needed.
- Asking for a calm adult to come out so that you can do some problem solving together.
- Taking five or ten minutes to help her contain the emotion and making sure that the person is safe, then letting her know when and how you can help more specifically.
- Speaking softly so as not to increase her anxiety.
- Encouraging her to breathe deeply.
- Remembering to either sit down or stand in a nonthreatening stance so as not to trigger her further.
- Calling the therapist.
- Calling 911 or going to the emergency room if she is threatening to commit suicide. (This behavior is different from self-mutilation, which is often manageable. A good resource for learning about self-mutilation is *The Scarred Soul: Understanding and Ending Self-Inflicted Violence*, by Tracy Alderman.)

Safety is extremely important to persons with DID. In the therapy situation, it is important to understand that the person with DID may do a quick scan of the office each session to make sure nothing has changed since the last session. He might also ask questions from time to time for reassurance that you are not angry with him or planning to leave. Sometimes the questions might actually be coming from another part, although you are not aware of it, so it is usually best to simply answer them or explore their meanings in as calm and reassuring a manner as possible. People with DID can also be easily startled. Even if you move to do something as benign as turning on a fan, calmly state what you are going to do beforehand. It is important for partners also to understand these issues. You might do playful things with the host, but then a child ego state appears and what was playful has now become frightening. You certainly cannot predict every circumstance, but if your partner reacts to something with a startled or fearful response, simply respect it and tone down your own behavior without making it personal.

It is important to try consciously to predict situations in which the person with DID is likely to be triggered so that a joint decision about how to handle things can be made. Prediction is true for therapy situations as well. Of course, this information comes to light through experience, so the process is ongoing. Figure 10.1 shows the process for self-care, and Figure 10.2 is an example of an emotional management plan to work on together.

Other topics to discuss include when touch is and is not okay. Some survivors are frightened by touch when they are experiencing strong emotion because it reminds them of abusive experiences in the past. Anger and anxiety are two emotions important to address. Self-soothing techniques are generally helpful in the case of anxiety. Anger can be less predictable because it can turn so quickly to rage. Rage is often related to survival instincts. Even though current conflicts are not likely to be life and death situations, they can feel that way to the person with DID. It is best to let the anger ride its course as long as neither you nor the other person is in any danger. In therapy, rage can occur when the therapist says something he considers to be neutral or matter of fact and it triggers something internally for the client (typically shame.) Being able to note patterns in the individual's responses is helpful in determining how to manage them.

We must all know our needs to develop a self-care plan, even if it will have only a slight positive impact in our life.

List your needs. _____
(Be sure to consider the mental/emotional/physical/spiritual categories of need.)

How can these needs be met? _____

Meeting needs will require at least two approaches:

What are you committing yourself to doing?
_____

What will you ask others to assist you in accomplishing?
_____

My weekly schedule is:

Monday_____

Tuesday_____

Wednesday_____

Thursday_____

Friday_____

Saturday_____

Sunday_____

What will it take for me to accomplish the following?

Consistently doing self-care_____

Resiliency_____

Focus_____

Energy_____

Competency_____

Happiness_____

My schedule for reevaluation of this plan is _____

Figure 10.1 Self-Care Process

List fifteen self-care strategies without any duplications in the columns. A self-care strategy is anything that makes one feel better about himself or herself that does not infringe on others or create any unsafe situation for anyone.

Mental	Emotional/Spiritual	Physical
_____	_____	_____
_____	_____	_____
_____	_____	_____
_____	_____	_____
_____	_____	_____
_____	_____	_____
_____	_____	_____
_____	_____	_____
_____	_____	_____
_____	_____	_____
_____	_____	_____
_____	_____	_____
_____	_____	_____

From Rick Ritter, MSW, LCSW, Certified Traumatologist. Used by permission.

Figure 10.2 Self-Care Plan

Doing so together is helpful in increasing awareness on the part of the dissociator. It also helps increase intimacy in the relationship, be it with a therapist, partner, or friend.

SELF-CARE

Setting clear boundaries and knowing useful soothing techniques are essential parts of navigating the rough waters of DID, but they are not enough. As a significant person in the life of someone with DID, you cannot be present in her life without first showing up for your own in a meaningful and fulfilling way.

Therapists can help themselves, and ultimately their clients, by modeling good boundaries and by continually assessing their own stress levels and responding accordingly. A backup therapist can help. A backup therapist can function in various ways. He might see the client from time to time to work on specific issues with which you do not feel competent. He might serve more as a consultant who meets with you and your client when you feel stuck in therapy or find yourselves caught in a power struggle that simply will not resolve itself. Or, he may simply provide coverage for you when you are away from the office. On the positive side, having a backup therapist means you are getting another opinion about the direction of treatment, and you know your client will be safe when you are away because she will have access to someone she knows and with whom she has already worked. The danger of having a backup therapist is the possibility of triangulation or splitting if the client becomes angry with one therapist and goes to the other. This danger is easily remedied through open communication and by allowing clients to express their feelings without judgment. It also means, however, that the therapists will not discuss each other with the client; the focus is on the client's experience and how it relates to the overall therapy. The client can learn more direct ways of communication and, when more than one therapist is involved, can learn how to ask for help, an important life skill.

The reality for some therapists is that they cannot have an entire caseload of clients with DID because it feels too demanding. For some, this extends to trauma clients in general. For other therapists, this is not even an issue. Do not judge your abilities as a therapist according to the decisions you make regarding caseload. Some therapists are able to see ten clients a week, others see thirty. Some see all trauma clients, others like to see clients with a variety of issues. The more experienced you become as a therapist, the more you will be able to determine with whom you most enjoy working and with whom you are most effective. If you pay attention to your inner preferences, you will be happier and will have more energy when you do focus on trauma work.

Other helpful activities for therapists include attending consultation groups with other professionals and accessing supervision with someone specializing in dissociative disorders. Many therapists also seek out their own therapy to safeguard against the possibility of having their own issues contaminate the therapy with their clients. Individual therapy can help with managing stress and resolving personal issues unrelated to the DID work you do. It can also help you work through any "compassion fatigue" you might experience as a result of listening to stories of child abuse and other kinds of trauma day in and day out.

In addition, each of us (friend, family member, or therapist) must create our own bag of destressing tricks to pull out on especially difficult days. What will you put in yours? Take a minute to brainstorm, remembering to include both solitary activities and time with family and friends.

A sense of humor is a great asset in just about any situation. A therapist who has a good sense of humor not only helps himself but his clients as well. Modeling humor is an effective way of teaching emotional management and self-nurturing. As your own survival technique, however, humor can manifest itself in various ways. Not only do you need a bag of destressing tricks, but you also need a treasure chest packed full of humor nuggets. The ability to laugh in the midst of stressful situations is a precious commodity.

Flexibility is another important ingredient to have when dealing with stress. A relationship with someone who has DID can be somewhat unpredictable at times. Moods can change quite abruptly, and you can be left feeling confused and thrown off balance. For the therapist, flexibility can be practiced by going with the client wherever it is they need to go during the session, as long as safety limits are understood and respected. It means being willing to set plans aside to address something that needs more immediate attention. It also means exercising the ability to flow with unexpected changes in mood and behavior in the client rather than ending up in a power struggle.

If you are a friend or family member of a person with DID, flexibility might mean a willingness to deal with a child part that is feeling scared right before you walk into a social gathering. Or, it might mean going someplace alone because your partner is not feeling up to dealing with the situation. In terms of your own happiness, though, it is about cultivating flexibility as a state of heart and mind. Are you willing to create a life for yourself that is not defined by dissociation? If so, you will feel less controlled when those issues do emerge.

Related to this discussion is an accepting and nonjudgmental stance regarding the relationship, something you will need to practice in all areas of your life to be effective. It is about living your life mindfully, with an awareness and attention to what is occurring in the present moment as opposed to a need to project and control what will happen in the future. This stance frees up both people in the relationship to feel as if they can be more genuine in the way they interact with each other.

Also, if you live with someone who has DID, it is important that you have your own interests and friends. As with any relationship, changing your life completely to accommodate the other person ultimately leads to disaster. You will have friends in common, of course, but do not think you have to define yourself according to the other person. You will be happier if you walk through life together rather than with one of you taking responsibility for the other. As discussed earlier in this chapter, honest communication is necessary when you are involved with someone with DID. This important part of any relationship is vital when dissociation is a part of the picture, because trust, abandonment, and attachment issues are at the core of the dissociator's life experience. One way to communicate honestly is by learning effective communication skills and ways of resolving conflicts. (See Figure 10.3.)

You can learn communication and conflict resolution skills through workshops, through couples therapy, or by reading any of the myriad self-help books written on the topic of communication. Learning about DID together is also a way of bolstering communication and emotional intimacy. Going to a support group for partners of persons with DID will help you better understand how your partner experiences life. It will also provide you with a way of dealing with your own relationship issues and a method of managing stressors that are a part of the relationship.

Living with someone who has DID can be difficult. If you are committed to the relationship, you are going to witness a lot of pain that you are not able to stop, which creates suffering of your own. It can be lonely sometimes, because out of respect for your partner you cannot automatically share her dissociation with others. In the same vein, you may feel fearful about sharing your experience because people may not understand. Worse yet, they might judge you. When flashbacks occur, you can feel helpless. When switching happens, you might blame yourself for triggering your partner when in fact it

Communication Components

Your ideas, feelings, and activities provide the content for most of your conversations with others. In the case of DID, both internal and external experiences are involved.

1. The first step is to understand your own experience.
2. The second step is to learn to express your experience more fully and accurately.
3. The third step is to attempt to understand the experience of the person with whom you are communicating.

Conflict Resolution

1. Focus on the present.
2. Discuss one topic at a time.
3. Make clear, specific statements.
4. Avoid mind reading or speaking for the other person.
5. Ask and give feedback to avoid any misunderstandings.
6. Avoid labeling or blaming the other person.
7. Begin and end the discussion on a positive note.
8. Take ownership of your own feelings, without judging them as good or bad.
9. Work toward a win–win resolution.

Figure 10.3 Principles of Communication and Conflict Resolution

may have nothing to do with you. You may blame yourself for her mood swings, internalizing the rage as opposed to placing it where it belongs, in the past. You may feel a need to save her even though you know you cannot. It is important to remember that you did not cause the DID and you can not make it go away. Loving your partner is the best thing you can do. Rescuing her is only hurtful to both of you in the long run. Seriously consider joining a support group for partners or getting involved in an on-line chat room. Taking care of yourself will actually help your partner feel relieved that she does not have to take care of you, too. It also tells her you are interested in dealing with the dissociation. Pretending that the issue does not exist or that all your relationship problems are a result of your partner's DID will merely increase her shame.

The most difficult situation by far is how to maintain equality in a relationship where one of the partners is often in crisis. It can be helpful to start with the assumption that we are all dependent on each other to some degree. The goal, then, is to strive for healthy dependency. You might think about some of the ways that loving partners are dependent on each other:

- When one is ill, the other might take care of her.
- When one is sad, the other might comfort him.
- When one is extremely stressed, the other might take on more of the household responsibilities.

Start by brainstorming times that each of you might be dependent on the other, then discuss how you might meet those dependency needs in a healthy way. An example is given in Figure 10.4.

These ideas are not written in stone, but these types of exercises help open communication and better equip you to deal with stress when it comes knocking at your door.

In summary, if you take care of yourself, you will be in a better place to be in relationship with others. And, as long as we are alive, we will be in relationship to Self and others. We are interconnected beings who need each other. That is something to celebrate!

Experience of Dissociator	*Ways a Partner or Friend Can Help*
1. Feeling overwhelmed by stress.	1. We can talk about how to divide responsibilities.
2. Switching to a younger part.	2. I can sit with you and listen until you feel safe.
3. A visit from my family.	3. I can help with the prep work and some of the entertaining so that it doesn't all fall on you.

Experience of Nondissociator	*Ways a Partner or Friend Can Help*
1. Conflict with a friend.	1. I can listen to you and just be supportive.
2. Work stress.	2. I can listen and take on some of your share of the responsibilities for the next week.
3. Severe case of the flu.	3. I'll pamper you as much as you want with chicken soup, runs to the drugstore, and so forth.

Experience of Dissociator	*Ways a Partner or Friend Can Help*
1.	1.
2.	2.
3.	3.
4.	4.
5.	5.

Experience of Nondissociator	*Ways a Partner or Friend Can Help*
1.	1.
2.	2.
3.	3.
4.	4.
5.	5.

Figure 10.4 Ways of Meeting Interdependency Needs

Epilogue

This book offers basic information to dissociators and the significant people in their lives about the understanding and management of DID. An equally important purpose of the book is to help those of you who dissociate regularly to begin to think about what that means to you and your life. Increased knowl-

[portions of text obscured by an insert]

always an important first step in making decisions about
the various issues in our lives. Another impor-
for those with dissociative identity disorder,
arn to relate to self and others in a more
ne that this book has given you some
begin to do just that. It is also im-
changes in your life at your own
ot increased unnecessarily. Use
o think about the information
book.

- The   can apply to my life as a
  result
- One th   nd or family member
  since re
- The new   e with my
  therapist a
- My immed
- My goals for   e . . .
- I will share the   people: . . .

Appendix A
Treatment Programs

Sometimes outpatient therapy is not enough. At times, it is ideal for a primary therapist and client to work her to access inpatient or residential treatment that will be priate and helpful. It is also preferable for dissociative s to be hospitalized in facilities that offer trauma-based pro- specifically tailored to address the issues associated with iation. This appendix is not meant to be a comprehensive he programs listed here, however, are ones that are well ones I have personally researched, or ones recommended y colleagues in the field of dissociation. The information subject to change at any given time, and therapists and should contact programs personally to determine their iateness for a specific individual. If you have difficulty in g a suitable program, contact the International Society for the Study of Dissociation (ISSD) at 847-480-0899 or by E-mail at issd@ issd. org, for a referral.

Center for Emotional Trauma Recovery at Lake Chelan
Lake Chelan Community Hospital
P.O. Box 908
Chelan, WA 98816
Phone: 800-233-0045
Description: This program offers short-term inpatient care for people with posttraumatic and dissociative disorders. According to the center's brochure, the therapeutic goal of this program is

to promote healing and recovery through interventions that complement the outpatient therapy of patients. Treatment is delivered by a multidisciplinary team, and trauma issues are addressed.

Forest View Trauma Program
1055 Medical Park Drive SE
Grand Rapids, MI 49546-3671
Phone: 800-949-8439
Web site: www.forestviewhospital.com
Description: This program provides an integrated approach to treating trauma with a goal of improving functioning and improving symptoms. It is identical to the Timberlawn Trauma Program described below.

Life Healing Center
P.O. Box 6758
Santa Fe, NM 87502
Phone: 800-989-7406
E-mail: lhc@life-healing.com
Web site: www.life-healing.com
Description: The Life Healing Center is a residential facility specializing in the treatment of emotional trauma. It also provides continuing care for chemical dependency and eating disorders. The center is appropriate for clients needing an intense and structured therapy environment and for dissociative clients who require self-management skills. The program addresses such issues as affective dysregulation, dissociative symptoms, posttraumatic reactions, and coping mechanisms such as self-injury, eating disorders, and chemical dependency that often accompany trauma. The center provides twenty-four-hour staff coverage with a therapist/client ratio of one to three. Both individual therapy and group therapy

are provided as well as twelve-step meetings when appropriate. Bodywork, an important component of trauma therapy, is also available through this program.

Masters and Johnson Trauma Unit

River Oaks Hospital
1525 River Oaks Road W.
New Orleans, LA 70123
Phone: 800-366-1740

Description: This program offers individual, group, and expressive therapies as well as education that helps clients address strong emotions and maladaptive thinking and behavior styles that are trauma based. It addresses dissociation by using a grief model that addresses core trauma issues.

McLean Dissociative Disorders and Trauma Program

115 Mill Street
Belmont, MA 02478
Phone: Women's Program: 617-855-2346 or 617-855-2761
Phone: Dissociative Disorders Partial Hospital Program:
    617-855-2173
Web site: www.mcleanhospital.org

Description: The Dissociative Disorders and Trauma Program at McLean Hospital treats adults with various difficulties related to past trauma. The emphasis is on the overall functioning of the individual. Various levels of care are available, including inpatient hospitalization, partial hospital services, and outpatient groups. The Dissociative Disorders Program staff has specialized training in dealing with the needs of trauma survivors and dissociative symptoms. The Women's Treatment Program also addresses trauma issues, but in a women-only setting.

National Treatment Center for Trauma Stabilization and Resolution

Del Amo Hospital
23700 Camino Del Sol
Torrance, CA 90505
Phone: 800-533-5266
Description: This program was created for the purpose of trauma stabilization and resolution. Treatment is based on the trauma model and uses cognitive therapies in the context of individual and group experiences.

New Life Treatment Centers

570 Glenneyre, Suite 107
Laguna Beach, CA 92651 (with several locations nationwide)
Phone: 800-639-5433
Description: This program is Christian based, which is important to some clients. The literature states that it treats the body, mind, and spirit by using biblical concepts as a foundation. It is not apparent from its literature, however, whether it specializes in the treatment of trauma, which would be important to explore with the treatment staff when considering a referral.

Psychiatric Institute of Washington

4228 Wisconsin Avenue, NW
Washington, DC 20016
Phone: 202-965-8400
Web site: www.psychinstitute.com
Description: The posttraumatic and dissociative disorders program provides short-term treatment and offers rapid stabilization and training in self-management skills. Treatment is provided through inpatient, partial hospitalization, or intensive outpatient programming.

Sheppard Pratt Health System
6501 North Charles Street
Baltimore, MD 21285
Phone: 410-938-5000
E-mail: info@sheppardpratt.org
Web site: www.sheppardpratt.org
Description: A continuum of care for trauma disorders that includes both inpatient and outpatient services is offered. The inpatient program teaches grounding and containment skills for dissociative clients. It offers individual, group, and family therapy as well as assessments for other conditions, such as substance abuse and eating disorders. The day hospital provides a structured environment for patients who are making the transition from hospitalization. The Center for Trauma Assessment offers structured diagnostic interviews and psychological assessments and a child and adolescent component for treating trauma-based disorders. Education is available for mental health professionals specializing in the treatment of trauma-related disorders.

Timberlawn Trauma Center
4600 Samuell Boulevard
Dallas, TX 75228
Phone: 800-426-4944
Description: This program describes itself as being dedicated to the treatment of survivors of psychological trauma who have a trauma-related disorder. The program offers both individual and group therapy, including trauma education, cognitive therapy, role training, and expressive activities. It also provides education for mental health professionals who treat trauma-based disorders.

University Behavior Center
250 Discovery Drive
Orlando, FL 32826
Phone: 407-281-7000
Description: This center is a residential treatment program for adolescent females recovering from trauma. The foundation of the program is the belief that healing and growth are directly related to an increase in self-awareness and knowledge. The program includes an initial assessment and stabilization phase, a working phase that addresses the trauma, and a resolution phase that focuses on integration of the previous phases.

Resratix B
Resources

NEWSLETTERS

First Person Plural
P.O. Box 1309, Wolverhampton
WV6 9XY, United Kingdom
E-mail: fpplural@aol.com
Description: The major plus for this newsletter is that it includes
book reviews and fun pages for child parts. Some of the material
in the sample issue is so personal that it can be hard to relate
to, but sometimes that may be what clients with DID are
looking for.

Many Voices
P.O. Box 2639
Cincinnati, OH 45201-2639
Description: This magazine is very well done and offers good information about dissociation. The majority of the information is
contributed by readers and often includes artwork as well. An
important component of this publication is the therapists' page,
which offers information and advice regarding dissociation.

NEEDID Voices
(For Individuals Healing from Dissociative Disorders and
Their Supporters)
NEEDID Support Network
P.O. Box 784
South Hadley, MA 01075
E-mail: NEEDID1@yahoo.com
Web site: http://www.needid.bizland.com
Description: This newsletter is written by and for individuals with
DID or other dissociative disorders, as well as the support people
in their lives. The list of past topics is impressive and includes such
things as therapy goals and methods and alternatives to disso-
ciating and traumatic thinking. One sample issue was very bal-
anced and included a fun page, which can be important to DID
adults who also experience child states. This publication accepts
submissions for articles, other writings, art, and cartoons from individuals living with dissociation, their support people, and professionals. It is published bimonthly, and yearly subscriptions are $36.

Survivorship
3181 Mission, #139
San Francisco, CA 94110
E-mail: info@survivorship.org
Web site: www.survivorship.org
Description: This magazine is very informative, although it tends to
focus on ritual abuse, which can be triggering for some people.
One special thing about this publication is the supplementary
piece, entitled "The Lifeboat," written especially for child parts.
"Littles," who are readers, contribute to this magazine with letters,
poetry, artwork, stories, and activities. This publication can also
be accessed on-line.

GENERAL RESOURCES

Center for Mindful Living
3206 Holmes Avenue
Minneapolis, MN 55408
Phone: 612-825-7658
Description: This center offers an eight-week course on mindfulness based on the Jon Kabat-Zinn program for stress management. The center also offers the same course tailored to meet the needs of mental health professionals.

Hazelden Foundation
P.O. Box 11
Center City, MN 55012-0011
Phone: 651-213-4225
Web site: www.hazelden.org
Description: This inpatient treatment facility for alcohol and drug addiction pioneered the model of care most widely used in the treatment of addiction, with satellite locations across the country. Ask about its treatment for dual diagnosis.

Renfrew Center
7700 Renfrew Lane
Coconut Creek, FL 33073
Phone: 800-736-3739
Description: Renfrew is best known for its work with eating disorders, but it has expanded to include a more comprehensive treatment program, which could be helpful for a trauma survivor who also suffers from an eating disorder. Renfrew also has a location in Pennsylvania.

Women for Sobriety, Inc.
P.O. Box 618
Quakertown, PA 18951
Phone: 215-536-8026
Description: This organization provides an alternative to AA for women offering meetings, pen pal programs, newsletters, and recovery literature.

ORGANIZATIONS RELATED TO TRAUMA AND DISSOCIATION

Cavalcade Productions
P.O. Box 2480
Nevada City, CA 95959
Phone: 800-345-5530
E-mail: cavpro@nccn.net
Web site: www.pacific.net/~cavideo/index.html
Description: Cavalcade supplies training videos for therapists and trauma survivors.

Colin Ross Institute
1701 Gateway, Suite 349
Richardson, TX 75080
Phone: 972-918-9588
E-mail: rossinst@rossinst.com
Web site: www.rossinst.com
Description: This institute provides training videos for therapists as well as current information regarding the treatment of trauma.

International Society for the Study of Dissociation (ISSD)
60 Revere Drive, Suite 500
Northbrook, IL 60062
Phone: 847-480-0899
E-mail: issd@issd.org
Web site: www.issd.org
Description: ISSD is an organization for professionals in the field of dissociation. It provides information and offers therapy referrals to individuals seeking to deal with trauma and dissociation issues. It also provides an excellent reference on DID treatment guidelines.

International Society for Traumatic Stress Studies (ISTSS)
60 Revere Drive, Suite 500
Northbrook, IL 60062
Phone: 847-480-9028
E-mail: istss@istss.org
Web site: www.istss.org
Description: ISTSS is a professional organization that provides information regarding trauma in general as well as therapy referrals. It also provides information on PTSD treatment guidelines.

Sidran Foundation and Press
200 East Joppa Road, Suite 207
Towson, MD 21286
Phone: 410-825-8888
E-mail: sidran@sidran.org
Web site: www.sidran.org
Description: This nonprofit organization provides both education and advocacy related to trauma issues. Call for a catalog of products, including an excellent brochure on DID.

Trauma Center
14 Fordham Road
Allston, MA 02134
Phone: 617-782-6460
E-mail: moreinfo@traumacenter.org
Web site: www.traumacenter.org
Description: This center provides training, consultation, and education for professionals; research information; and links to sites that deal with the issue of trauma. The medical director is Bessel van der Kolk, M.D., an expert in the field of psychological trauma.

BOOKS OF INTEREST

The number of books available on trauma and dissociation are too numerous to mention. A few of the better-known books in the field are listed below. Others are listed because clients have found them to be especially helpful or because they reflect a view of trauma and dissociation found to be particularly useful in addressing the issues most often associated with dissociation. These suggestions should not be considered a comprehensive listing, but can be considered a good introduction to the literature associated with trauma and dissociation, specifically DID. The books are listed according to primary audiences; many, however, are useful to anyone interested in DID. Therapists and other support people can greatly benefit from information about what it is like to live with DID.

Books of Interest to
Children, Child Parts, and Grown-Ups, Too

The Giver, Lois Lowry, Bantam, 1993

Horton Hears a Who, Theodor Geisel (Dr. Seuss), Random House, 1982.

Love You Forever, Robert Munsch, Firefly Books, 1986

My Many-Colored Days, Theodor Geisel (Dr. Seuss), Knopf, 1996.

My Mom Is Different, Deborah Sessions, Sidran Press, 1994.

Oh, The Places You'll Go, Theodor Geisel (Dr. Seuss), Random House, 1990.

The Velveteen Rabbit, Margery Williams, Henry Holt, 1983.

Wemberly Worried, Kevin Henkes, Green Willow Books, 2000.

The Paper Bag Princess, Robert Munsch, Annick Press, 1980

Books of Interest to
Individuals Living with DID

Amongst Ourselves: A Self-Help Guide to Living with Dissociative Identity Disorder, Karen Marshall and Tracey Alderman, New Harbinger, 1998.

I Can't Get Over It: A Handbook for Trauma Survivors, Aphrodite Matsakis, New Harbinger, 1996.

Living with Your Selves: A Survival Manual for People with Multiple Personalities, Sandra J. Hocking, Launch Press, 1992.

The Magic Daughter, Jane Phillips, Penguin, 1995.

Managing Ourselves: Building a Community of Caring, Elizabeth E. Powers, Power and Associates, 1992.

Multiple Personality Disorder from the Inside Out, Barry M. Cohen, Norton, 1995.

Outgrowing the Pain, Eliana Gil, Dell Publishing, 1983.

The Silver Boat, Ann Adams, Behavioral Science Center, Inc. Publications, 1990.

The Silver Boat II, Ann Adams, Behavioral Science Center, Inc. Publications, 1994.

United We Stand: A Book for People with Multiple Personalities, Eliana Gil, Launch Press, 1990.

Books of Interest to Support People

Allies in Healing, Laura Davis, HarperCollins, 1991.

Ghosts in the Bedroom: A Guide for Partners of Incest Survivors, Ken Graber, Health Communications, 1991.

Someone I Know Has Multiple Personalities: A Book for Significant Others—Friends, Family, and Caring Professionals, Sandra J. Hocking, Launch Press, 1994.

Books of Interest to Therapists

Adult Survivors of Child Sexual Abuse, Christine Courtois, Families Intl., 1993

Affect Regulation and the Origin of the Self: The Neurobiology of Emotional Development, Allan Schore, Laurence Erlbaum Assoc., 1999

Assessment and Treatment of Multiple Personality and Dissociation, J. P. Block, Professional Resource Press, 1991.

The Body Remembers: The Psychobiology of Trauma and Trauma Treatment, Babette Rothschild, W.W. Norton, 2000

Clinical Perspectives on Multiple Personality Disorder, Richard P. Kluft and Catherine G. Fine, eds., American Psychiatric Press, 1993.

Countertransference and the Treatment of Trauma, Constance Dalenberg, American Psychological Association, 2000

The Developing Mind, Daniel Siegel, Guilford Press, 1999

Diagnosis and Treatment of Multiple Personality, Frank Putnam, Foundations of Modern Psychiatry, 1989.

Dissociative Identity Disorder: Diagnosis, Clinical Features, and Treatment of Multiple Personality, Colin Ross, Wiley, 1996.

Dissociation in Children and Adolescents: A Developmental Perspective, Frank Putnam, Guilford Press, 1997

EMDR in the Treatment of Adults Abused as Children, Laurel Parnell, Norton, 1999.

Effective Treatments for PTSD, Edna Foa (Ed.), Guilford Press, 2000

Eye Movement Desensitization and Reprocessing, Francine Shapiro, Guilford Press, 1995.

The Family Inside: Working with the Multiple, Doris Bryant, Judy Kessler, and Linda Shirar, Norton, 1992.

Healing the Incest Wound: Adult Survivors in Therapy, Christine Courtois, W.W. Norton, 1988

Measurement of Stress, Trauma, and Adaptation, B. Hudnall Stamm (Ed.), Sidran Press, 1996.

Molecules of Emotion, Candace Pert, Scribner, 1997

The Mosaic Mind, Goulding and Schwartz, W.W. Norton, 1995

Multiple Personality and Dissociation, 1791–1992: A Complete Bibliography, Carole Goettman, George B. Greaves, and Philip M. Coons, eds., Sidran, 1994.

Not Trauma Alone: Therapy for Child Abuse Survivors in Family and Social Context, Steven Gold, Brunner/Routledge, 2000

Post-Traumatic Stress Disorder: The Victim's Guide to Healing and Recovery, Raymond Flannery, Crossroad, 1992

Rebuilding Shattered Lives, J. Chu, Wiley, 1998.

Sexual Abuse and Eating Disorders, Mark Schwartz and Leigh Cohn, Brunner Mazel, 1996.

Trauma and Recovery, Judith Herman, Basic Books, 1992.

Trauma and the Therapist, Laurie Pearlman and Karen W. Saakvitne, Norton, 1995.

Treating Dissociative Identity Disorder, Irvin Yalom and James Spira, eds., Jossey-Bass, 1996.

Books of General Interest

The Depression Sourcebook, Brian P. Quinn, Contemporary Books/McGraw-Hill, 1998.

The Eating Disorder Sourcebook, Carolyn Costin, Contemporary Books/McGraw-Hill, 1996.

Eight Weeks to Optimum Health, Andrew Weil, Ballantine, 1997.

Emotional Intelligence, Daniel Goleman, Bantam, 1995

Full Catastrophe Living, Jon Kabat-Zinn, Dell Publishing, 1990.

Peace Is Every Step: The Path of Mindfulness in Everyday Life, T. N. Hanh, Bantam, 1991.

Reclaiming Our Bodies, Rebecca L. Zuckweiler, Parkside Publishing, 1993.

Touching Peace: Practicing the Art of Mindful Living, T. N. Hanh, Parallax Press, 1992.

Waking the Tiger, Peter Levine, North Atlantic Books, 1997

Workbooks

The Anger Control Workbook, Matthew McKay, New Harbinger, 2000

The Anger Workbook, Les Carter and Frank Minirth, Thomas Nelson Publishers, 1993.

The Anxiety and Phobia Workbook, Edmund Bourne, New Harbinger, 1995.

The Courage to Heal Workbook, Laura Davis, HarperCollins, 1990.

Growing Beyond Abuse, S. Nestingen, Omni Recovery, Inc., 1990.

The Emotional Freedom Workbook, Stephen Arterburn, Thomas Nelson, 1997

Healing the Trauma of Abuse, Mary Ellen Copeland, New Harbinger, 2000

Imaging Your Self, K. Giguere, Horizons, 1994.
Mind Over Mood, Dennis Greenberger, Guilford Press, 1995

The Relaxation and Stress Reduction Workbook, Matthew McKay, New Harbinger

Sark's Journal and Playbook, Celestial Arts, 1993

Thoughts and Feelings: Taking Control of Your Moods and Your Life, Matthew McKay, New Harbinger, 1997

INTERNET SITES

Internet sites are too numerous to mention, but each site listed here is one I personally visited. It is important to remember that in the case of chat rooms and bulletin boards, you cannot be 100 percent sure with whom you are communicating. Consequently, it is important to keep yourself safe by guarding personal information such as home addresses, phone numbers, and even your real name. It would also be inappropriate, in my opinion, for a child part to be engaging in Internet activities alone because it sets the stage for possible re-traumatization. Generally, Internet discussions are best left to adult parts with good decision-making skills and an ability to manage triggers. If you are unsure about the suitability of a site, be sure to discuss it with your therapist. Internet sites are constantly changing, and the material below cannot be guaranteed to be completely accurate at any given time.

Absolute Authority
www.absoluteauthority.com/DID_MPD/
This is a comprehensive site to visit and find information regarding dissociation, with links to many other sites appropriate to dissociators, concerned others, and therapists.

Amongst Others
www.foxfiremad.com/amongst
This site provides information for patients and significant others regarding dissociation. It is a restricted list, which is helpful in terms of safety. The site includes a link to **Healing Rainbows**, a Web ring for partners and friends of multiples.

BPD Sanctuary

www.mhsanctuary.com/borderline/

This site offers valuable information for borderline individuals, therapists, and other concerned persons as well regarding borderline personality disorder.

Children of Multiplicity

www.survivorship.org

This site offers general information for multiples and focuses heavily on ritual abuse. It is, for the most part, a member-only site. You can access the *Survivorship* magazine on-line at this site.

David Baldwin's Trauma Pages

www.trauma-pages.com

This is considered the premier trauma site on the Web. It provides accurate and up-to-date information on issues related to trauma and is appropriate for anyone interested in learning more about the topic.

Empty Memories

www.utopis.knoware.nl

This site is very well done and inviting. It is one of my favorites on the Web in terms of its appropriateness for anyone who is looking for good information about trauma and dissociation. The pages are very inviting, creatively done, and available in both Dutch and English.

4therapy

www.4therapy.com

This site is a therapist locator. Information and articles about mental health issues are also provided.

Healing Hopes
www.healinghopes.org
This site serves as a support forum for trauma survivors, especially those with DID. It offers a newsroom with an on-line newsletter, a library containing information about DID, chat rooms, message boards, and links to Web rings.

Mental Health Matters
www.mental-health-matters.com
This site provides information and resources for professionals, consumers, and families. You can subscribe to a mental health matters newsletter via E-mail as well.

Mosaic Minds
www.mosaicminds.org
This site offers seventeen message forums for people affected by dissociation, a creativity corner, a reading room, a bookstore, and tips for managing triggers.

MPD Spouses, a Yahoo Club
clubs.yahoo.com/clubs/mpdspouses
This site provides a forum where support people can go to talk about how their lives are affected by being in relationships with persons with DID.

Multiple Personality
www.multiple-personality.com
This site was created by someone with a diagnosis of DID and offers current information on the topic of dissociation.

NEEDID Support Network

www.needid.bizland.com

This site offers resources for individuals who are dissociative as well as their significant others. It also publishes a bimonthly newsletter.

Pat McClendon's Clinical Social Work

www.clinicalsocialwork. com

This site offers an array of information on topics ranging from abuse to addictions to therapy approaches to dissociation. It also provides many links to sites related to these topics. It is great for professionals, but is also helpful for anyone who is looking for good information on mental health issues.

PILOTS Database

www.ncptsd.org

This site is an extensive trauma database for therapists.

Significant Other's Guide to DID

www.op.net/~jeffv/so1.htm

Information about being a partner to someone with DID is on this site. The guide is available to download and contains lots of practical information and humor.

Wounded Healer Journal and Message Forum

www.twhj.com

An excellent site for therapists who have experienced trauma of their own. It also has a forum for support people involved with someone who has a dissociative disorder.

Notes

CHAPTER ONE

1. R. J. Loewenstein, "Multiple Personality Disorder: A Continuing Challenge," *Psychiatry Review 2* (1989) 1–2. There are many estimates regarding the prevalence of DID; most are in the 1 to 5 percent range, with higher percentages found among psychiatric populations.

2. K. Steele and J. Colrain, "Abreactive Work with Sexual Abuse Survivors: Concepts and Techniques," in *The Sexually Abused Male: Vol. 2: Application of Treatment Strategies*, ed. M. A. Hunter (Lexington, Mass.: Lexington Books, 1990).

3. American Psychiatric Association, *Diagnostic and Statistical Manual of Mental Disorders*, 4th ed. (Washington, D.C.: American Psychiatric Association, 1994).

4. J. Herman, *Trauma and Recovery* (New York: Basic Books, 1992); J. Watkins and H. Watkins, "The Theory and Practice of Ego State Therapy." In *Short Term Approaches to Psychotherapy*, ed. H. Grayson (New York: Human Sciences Press, 1979).

5. Watkins and Watkins, "The Theory and Practice of Ego State Therapy"; E. Weiss, *The Structure and Dynamic of the Human Mind* (New York: Grune and Stratton, 1960); P. Federn, in *Ego Psychology and the Psychoses*, ed. E. Weiss (New York: Basic Books, 1952).

6. F. Putnam, *Diagnosis and Treatment of Multiple Personality Disorder* (New York: Guilford Press, 1989).

7. B. O'Regan, "Multiple Personality—Mirrors of a New Mind," *Investigations* (Institute of Noetic Sciences), no. 3–4 (1985): 1–23.

8. B. Perry, "Neurodevelopment and Dissociation: Trauma and Adaptive Responses to Fear," presentation to the International Society for the Study of Dissociation conference, San Antonio (2000).

9. S. Roth and M. Friedman, eds., *Childhood Trauma Remembered* (Chicago: International Society for Traumatic Stress Studies).

10. Watkins and Watkins, "The Theory and Practice of Ego State Therapy."

11. B. van der Kolk, A. C. McFarlane, and L. Weisaeth, eds., *Traumatic Stress* (New York: Guilford Press, 1996).

12. B. van der Kolk, lecture on trauma and memory, Cape Cod Institute (1998).

CHAPTER TWO

1. J. Curtis, "DID as a Developmental Disorder: Therapeutic Implications," presentation to the International Society for the Study of Dissociation conference, San Antonio (2000); P. M. Barach, "Multiple Personality Disorder as an Attachment Disorder," *Dissociation* 4 (1991): 117–23; G. Liotti, "Disorganized/Disoriented Attachment in the Etiology of the Dissociative Disorders," *Dissociation* 5, no. 4 (1992): 196–204.

2. A. Maslow, *Toward a Psychology of Being* (New York: Van Nostrand, Reinhold (1968).

3. B. van der Kolk, lecture on trauma and memory; B. van der Kolk and R. Fisler, "Dissociation and the Fragmentary Nature of Traumatic Memories: Overview and Exploratory Study," *Journal of Traumatic Stress* 8, no. 4 (1995): 505–25.

4. F. Knopp and A. Benson, *A Primer on the Complexities of Traumatic Memory of Childhood Sexual Abuse* (Brandon, Vt.: Safer Society Press, 1996).

5. R. Karen, "Will Your Child Be Happy in Love?" *Child*, February 1995, 111–13.

6. B. James, "Long-Term Treatment for Children with Severe Trauma History," In *Handbook of Post-Traumatic Therapy* eds. M. B. Williams and J. F. Sommer (Westport, Conn.: Greenwood Press, 1994).

CHAPTER THREE

1. C. A. Ross, *Multiple Personality Disorder: Diagnosis, Clinical Features, and Treatment* (New York: John Wiley, 1989); Putnam, *Diagnosis and Treatment of Multiple Personality Disorder.*

2. Ross, *Multiple Personality Disorder.*

3. Ross, *Multiple Personality Disorder*; Putnam, *Diagnosis and Treatment of Multiple Personality Disorder.*

4. J. Chu, *Rebuilding Shattered Lives* (New York: John Wiley, 1998).

5. Herman, *Trauma and Recovery*; Ross, *Multiple Personality Disorder.* Many clinicians are beginning to treat disorders such as DID, BPD, and PTSD from a trauma model that emphasizes the treatment of the posttrauma symptoms more than the individual diagnosis.

6. Putnam, *Diagnosis and Treatment of Multiple Personality Disorder*; Ross, *Multiple Personality Disorder.*

7. E. Nijenhaus, *Somatoform Dissociation: Phenoma, Measurement, and Theoretical Issues* (Assen, The Netherlands: Van Gorcum, 1999).

8. Putnam, *Diagnosis and Treatment of Multiple Personality Disorder.*

9. R. B. Flannery, *Post-Traumatic Stress Disorder: The Victim's Guide to Healing and Recovery* (New York: Crossroad, 1992); M. Schwartz and L. Cohn, eds., *Sexual Abuse and Eating Disorders* (New York: Brunner/Mazel, 1996).

10. B. G. Braun, "The BASK Model of Dissociation," *Dissociation* 1, no. 2 (1988): 4–23.

11. B. van der Kolk, "The Body Keeps the Score: Memory and the Evolving Psychobiology of Post-Traumatic Stress," *Harvard Review Psychiatry* 1 (1994): 253–65.

12. Putnam, *Diagnosis and Treatment of Multiple Personality Disorder.*

13. Ross, *Multiple Personality Disorder.*

14. Nijenhuis, *Somatoform Dissociation.*

15. M. Steinberg, *Structured Clinical Interview for DSM-IV Dissociative Disorders Revised* (Washington, D.C.: American Psychiatric Press, 1994).

16. P. M. Coons and A. L. Sterne, "Initial and Follow-up Psychological Testing on a Group of Patients with Multiple Personality Disorder," *Psychological Reports* 58 (1986): 43–49; R. Solomon, "The Use of the MMPI with Multiple Personality Patients," *Psychological Reports* 53 (1983): 1004–6; E. L. Bliss, "A Symptom Profile of Patients with Multiple Personalities, Including MMPI Results," *Journal of Nervous and Mental Disease* 172 (1984): 197–202.

CHAPTER FOUR

1. R. Schwartz, "Our Multiple Selves: Applying Systems Theory to the Inner Family," *Family Therapy Networker* 11 (1987): 25–31, 80–83.

2. H. Watkins, "Ego-State Therapy: An Overview," *American Journal of Clinical Hypnosis* 35, no. 4 (1993): 232–40.

3. *Clinical Perspectives on Multiple Personality Disorder,* edited by R. P. Kluft and C. G. Fine (Washington, D.C.: American Psychiatric Press, 1993).

4. J. G. Watkins, *The Therapeutic Self* (New York: Human Sciences Press, 1978).

CHAPTER FIVE

1. G. Fraser, "The Dissociative Table Technique: A Strategy for Working with Ego States in Dissociative Disorders and Ego-State Therapy," *Dissociation* 4: 205–13.

2. C. Ross, "The Locus of Control Shift." Material from the Timberlawn trauma program directed by Colin Ross, M.D.

3. L. J. Dickstein, "Spouse Abuse and Other Domestic Violence," *Psychiatric Clinics of North America* 11, no. 4 (1998): 611–28.

CHAPTER SIX

1. I. D. Yalom, *The Theory and Practice of Group Psychotherapy*, 3d ed. (New York: Basic Books, 1985).

2. M. Linehan, *Skills Training Manual for Treating Borderline Personality Disorder* (New York: Guilford Press, 1993).

3. J. Kabat-Zinn, *Full Catastrophe Living: Using the Wisdom of Your Body and Mind to Face Stress, Pain, and Illness* (New York: Dell, 1990).

4. F. Shapiro, *Eye Movement Desensitization and Reprocessing* (New York: Guilford Press, 1995).

CHAPTER SEVEN

1. Many thanks to Dr. Tim Richardson for his help in putting this information together.

2. "Herbal Medicine," http://www.depression.com/health_library, 1999, (3 December 1999).

3. *Journal of Clinical Psychiatry* (1999) 60: 598–603.

4. Zeuss quoted in "Herbal Index," http:/www.onhealth.com/alternative/resources/herbs, 1999 (31 May 2000).

5. "Constituents of Essential Oil from Leaves of Liquid Ambar Styraciflual," *Planta Medica* 38 (1980): 79–85.

6. Albert (1994).

7. M. Torem, "Medications in the Treatment of Dissociative Identity Disorder," in *Treating Dissociative Identity Disorder* J. L. Spira and I. D. Yalom, eds. (San Francisco: Jossey-Bass, 1996).

Chapter Eight

1. Yalom, *The Theory and Practice of Group Psychotherapy.*

2. International Society for the Study of Dissociation, *Guidelines for Treatment* (Chicago: International Society for the Study of Dissociation, 1997).

3. J. Cameron, *The Artist's Way* (New York: G. P. Putnam's Sons, 1992).

Chapter Nine

1. Fraser, "The Dissociative Table Technique."

Bibliography

ALDERMAN, T. *The Scarred Soul: Understanding and Ending Self-Inflicted Violence.* Oakland, Calif: New Harbinger Publications, 1997.

AMERICAN PSYCHIATRIC ASSOCIATION. *Diagnostic and Statistical Manual of Mental Disorders,* 4th ed. Washington, D.C.: American Psychiatric Association, 1994.

BERGMANN, U. "Speculations on the Neurobiology of EMDR." *Traumatology* no. 1 (1998): 4; 4–16.

BLISS, E. L. "A Symptom Profile of Patients with Multiple Personalities, Including MMPI Results." *Journal of Nervous and Mental Disease* 4 (1984): 172, 197–202.

BLOCH, J. *Assessment and Treatment of Multiple Personality and Dissociative Disorders.* Sarasota, Fla.: Professional Resource Press, 1981.

BRAUN, B. G. "The BASK Model of Dissociation." *Dissociation* 1, no. 2 (1988): 4–23.

BRAUN, B. G., ed. *Treatment of Multiple Personality Disorder.* Washington, D.C.: American Psychiatric Press, 1986.

BRENDE, J. O. "Dissociative Disorders in Vietnam and Combat Veterans." *Journal of Contemporary Psychotherapy* 17 (1987): 77–86.

BRODAL, A. *Neurological Anatomy in Relation to Clinical Medicine,* 3rd ed. New York: Oxford University Press, 1980.

BRODAL, P. *The Central Nervous System: Structure and Function.* New York: Oxford University Press, 1992.

CHU, J. *Rebuilding Shattered Lives.* New York: John Wiley, 1998.

COONS, P. M., and A. L. STERNE, "Initial and Follow-Up Psychological Testing on a Group of Patients with Multiple Personality Disorder." *Psychological Reports* 58, (1986): 43–49.

DICKSTEIN, L. J. "Spouse Abuse and Other Domestic Violence." *Psychiatric Clinics of North America* 11, no. 4 (1988): 611–28.

ELCHISAK, MARY A. "Pharmacology." http://www.about.com/
    pharma. 1999. (2 December 1999).
FEDERN, P. *Ego Psychology and the Psychoses,* edited by E. Weiss.
    (New York: Basic Books, 1952).
FOX, I. "Attachment Parenting: What the Authorities Say."
    www.attachmentparenting.org (8 April 2000).
FRASER, G. A., "The Dissociative Table Technique: A Strategy for
    Working with Ego States in Dissociative Disorders and Ego-
    State Therapy." *Dissociation* 4, 205–13.
GILBERT, M. "Managing Stress: Pathways to Adaptation and
    Balance." Healthwell.com.http://www.healthwell.com/
    hnbreakthroughs (1999).
"Herbal Index." http:/onhealth.com/alternative/resources/herbs
    (1999).
"Herbal Medicine." http://www.depression.com/health_library
    (1999).
HERMAN, J. *Trauma and Recovery.* New York: Basic Books, 1992.
HOBSON, J. A., R. STICKGOLD, and E. PACE-SCHOTT, "The
    Neuropsychology of REM Sleep Dreaming." *Neuroreport* 9
    (1998): R1–R14.
HOCKING, S. J. *Living with Your Selves: A Survival Manual for
    People with Multiple Personalities.* Rockville, Md.: Launch Press,
    1992.
HOLT, D. "The Role of the Amygdala in Fear and Panic." http://
    serendip.brynmawr.edu (1998).
"Homeopathy." http://onhealth.com/alternative/resource (1999).
HUDSON, P. S. *Ritual Child Abuse.* Saratoga, Calif.: R & E Pub-
    lishers, 1991.
INTERNATIONAL SOCIETY FOR THE STUDY OF DISSOCIATION.
    Guidelines for Treatment. Chicago: Int. Society for the Study of
    Dissociation, 1997.
JANET, P. *The Major Symptoms of Hysteria.* New York: Macmillan,
    1907.
JONES, STANTON L., and R. E. BUTMAN, *Modern Psychotherapies.*
    Downers Grove, Ill.: InterVarsity Press, 1991.
KABAT-ZINN, J. *Full Catastrophe Living: Using the Wisdom of Your
    Body and Mind to Face Stress, Pain, and Illness.* New York: Dell,
    1990.

KAREN, R. "Will Your Child be Happy in Love?" *Child* (February 1995): 111–13.

KLUFT, R. P. "An Update on Multiple Personality Disorder." *Hospital and Community Psychiatry* 38 (1987): 363–73.

———. "Current Issues in Dissociative Identity Disorder." *Journal of Practical Psychiatry and Behavioral Health* 5 (1999): 3–19.

———. "The Psychoanalytic Psychotherapy of Dissociative Identity Disorder in the Context of Trauma Therapy." *Psychoanalytic Inquiry* 20, no. 2 (2000): 259–83.

———. "An Overview of the Psychotherapy of Dissociative Identity Disorder." *American Journal of Psychotherapy* 53 (2000): 289–319.

KNOPP, F. H., and A. R. BENSON. *A Primer on the Complexities of Traumatic Memory of Childhood Sexual Abuse*. Brandon, Vt.: Safer Society Press, 1996.

LINEHAN, M. *Skills Training Manual for Treating Borderline Personality Disorder*. New York: Guilford Press, 1993.

LOEWENSTEIN, R. J. "Multiple Personality Disorder: A Continuing Challenge." *Psychiatry Review* 2 (1989): 1–2.

MANN, J. J. "The Neurobiology of Suicide." 4, no. 1 (January 1998): 25–30. *Nature Medicine*. January 1998.

MAY, R., and I. YALOM, "Existential Psychotherapy," in *Current Psychotherapies*, edited by R. J. Corsini and D. Wedding. Itasca, Ill.: F. E. Peacock, 1989.

NADEL, L., and M. MOSCOVITCH. "Hippocampal Contributions to Cortical Plasticity." *Neuropharmacology* 37 (1998): 431–39.

NICHOLSON, B. "The Attachment Cycle." http://www.attachmentparenting.org. (8 April 2000)

NIJENJUIS, E.R.S. *Somatoform Dissociation: Phenoma, Measurement, and Theoretical Issues*. Assen, The Netherlands: Van Gorcum, 1999.

NORTH, C. S., ET AL. *Multiple Personalities, Multiple Disorders: Psychiatric Classification and Media Influence*. New York: Oxford University Press, 1993.

O'REGAN, B., ED. "Multiple Personality—Mirrors of a New Mind." *Investigations* (Institute of Noetic Sciences) 1, no. 3–4 (1985): 1–23.

PECK, M. S. *The Road Less Traveled.* New York: Touchstone Books, 1988.

PRINCE, M. *Dissociation of a Personality.* New York: Longman, Green, 1906.

PUTNAM, F. *Diagnosis and Treatment of Multiple Personality Disorder.* New York: Guilford Press, 1989.

REISER, M. *Memory in Mind and Brain: What Dream Imagery Reveals.* New Haven: Yale University Press, 1994.

ROSS, C. A. *Multiple Personality Disorder: Diagnosis, Clinical Features, and Treatment.* New York: John Wiley, 1989.

———. *Dissociative Identity Disorder: Diagnosis, Clinical Features, and Treatment of Multiple Personality.* New York: John Wiley, 1996.

ROSS, S., and M. FRIEDMAN, EDS. *Childhood Trauma Remembered.* Chicago: International Society for Traumatic Stress Studies.

SCHACTER, D. L., and E. TULVING. *Memory Systems.* Cambridge: MIT Press, 1994.

SCHIRALDI, G. R. *The Post-Traumatic Stress Disorder Sourcebook: A Guide to Healing, Recovery, and Growth.* Los Angeles: Lowell House, 2000.

SCHWARTZ, M., and L. COHN, EDS. *Sexual Abuse and Eating Disorders.* New York: Brunner/Mazel, 1996.

SCHWARTZ, R. C. "The Internal Family Systems Model." http:/www.internalfamilysystems.org/outline.htmp (14 January 2000).

———. "Our Multiple Selves: Applying Systems Theory to the Inner Family." *Family Therapy Networker* (1987): 11, 25–31, 80–83.

SHAPIRO, F. *Eye Movement Desensitization and Reprocessing.* New York: Guilford Press, 1995.

SOLOMON, R. "The Use of the MMPI with Multiple Personality Patients." *Psychological Reports* 53 (1983): 1004–6.

SPEIGEL, D. "Multiple Personality as a PTSD." *Psychiatric Clinics of North America* 7 (1984): 101–10.

SPIRA, J. L., and I. D. YALOM, EDS. *Treating Dissociative Identity Disorder.* San Francisco: Jossey-Bass, 1996.

STEELE, K., and J. COLRAIN. "Abreactive Work with Sexual Abuse Survivors: Concepts and Techniques." In *The Sexually Abused Male: Vol. 2: Application of Treatment Strategies*, edited by M. A. Hunter. Lexington, Mass.: Lexington Books, 1990.

STEINBERG, M. *Structured Clinical Interview for DSM-IV Dissociative Disorders Revised*. Washington, D.C.: American Psychiatric Press, 1994.

STICKGOLD, ET AL. "Sleep-Induced Changes in Associative Memory." *Journal of Cognitive Neuroscience* 11: 182–93.

TOREM, M. "Medications in the Treatment of Dissociative Identity Disorder." In *Treating Dissociative Identity Disorder*, edited by J. Spira and I. D. Yalom. San Francisco: Jossey-Bass, 1996.

VAN DER KOLK, B. A. "The Body Keeps the Score: Memory and the Evolving Psychobiology of Post-Traumatic Stress." *Harvard Review Psychiatry* 1 (1994): 253–65.

VAN DER KOLK, B. A., and R. FISLER. "Dissociation and the Fragmentary Nature of Traumatic Memories: Overview and Exploratory Study." *Journal of Traumatic Stress* 8, no. 4 (1995): 505–25.

VAN DER KOLK, B. A., A. C. MCFARLANE, and L. WEISAETH, EDS. *Traumatic Stress*. New York: Guilford Press, 1996.

WALKER, L. E. A. "Psychology and Violence Against Women." *American Psychologist* 44, no. 4 (1989): 695–702.

WATKINS, H. H. "Ego-State Therapy: An Overview." *American Journal of Clinical Hypnosis* 35, no. 4 (1993): 232–40.

WATKINS, J. G. *The Therapeutic Self*. New York: Human Sciences Press, 1978.

WATKINS, J. G, and H. H. WATKINS. "The Theory and Practice of Ego-State Therapy." In *Short-Term Approaches to Psychotherapy*. New York: Human Sciences Press, 1979.

———. "Ego-State Therapy in the Treatment of Dissociative Disorders." In *Clinical Perspectives on Multiple Personality Disorder*, edited by R. P. Kluft and C. G. Fine, American Psychiatric Press, Washington, D.C., 1993.

WEIL, A. *Eight Weeks to Optimum Health*. New York: Ballantine, 1997.

WEISS, E. *The Structure and Dynamics of the Human Mind*. New York: Grune and Stratton, 1960.

WILLIAMS, M. B., and J. F. SOMMER, EDS. *Handbook of Post-Traumatic Therapy.* Westport, Conn.: Greenwood Press, 1994.

WINSON, J. *Brain and Psyche: The Biology of the Unconscious.* New York: Doubleday/Anchor Press, 1985.

YALOM, I. D. *Existential Psychotherapy.* New York: Basic Books, 1980.

———. *The Theory and Practice of Group Psychotherapy,* 3d ed. New York: Basic Books, 1985.

Index